RETHiNK®

health

live younger longer

PAUL O'MAHONY & ANGELA FOSTER

RETHiNK® health

live younger longer

PAUL O'MAHONY & ANGELA FOSTER

Contents

Preface

"It's worse than I thought" were the Consultant's words as I walked back into his office after a CT scan for lung cancer. Immediately admitted into hospital as an emergency case, unable to collect my kids from school and explain to them what was going on, I was hooked up to intravenous drips and oxygen. It felt like a far cry from my former life as a successful corporate lawyer.

As a typical 'Type A' personality I was used to working hard and pushing through long nights and weekends of work to close multinational deals for big corporations. I loved the thrill of the deal and was driven by achieving success for myself and my high paying clients. Luxury vacations to tropical locations allowed me the time to catch up and reboot before then launching myself back into the corporate world. I felt invincible.

Life continued in the same vein for many years. It changed radically when after having my three children I was diagnosed with chronic depressive disorder and placed on bipolar medication under psychiatric care at the Priory Hospital.

In the early days after having kids I ignored the signs of postpartum depression. That was something that 'other women' experienced. I put it down to just being tired out, exhausted by the demands of looking after 3 children under 4 years old.

And so I pushed on. My hair started to fall out and I didn't feel like taking care of myself anymore, but I carried on regardless.

Behind the smiles and good morning pleasantries demanded by the school run was a growing darkness inside me that cloaked my every thought and action.

As the months and years went on, it felt like the sun didn't shine anymore. Even on the brightest and most glorious day everything still seemed numbingly grey.

With 3 different prescribed psychiatric medications, it still took 2 hours and repeated calls of "Mummy, please" from my four year old to rouse me from my slumber and drag me out of bed.

The days blurred into weeks and months.

"You need to be more compassionate with yourself" my therapist told me; "do less and ask for more help".

How could I possibly do less? Getting my eldest son to school on time was an impressive achievement during those dark days.

I was a mere shadow of the vibrant, happy and successful woman that I used to be and my mood had turned progressively darker. With the constant chatter in my head, thoughts of suicide seemed the only way to switch off my mind. And so the darkness continued, slowly drawing me further into the abyss until one spring day I developed a cough and a fever.

Dosing myself with the usual paracetamol and ibuprofen, I carried on until breathing became harder and the fever made it even more difficult to get out of bed. A chest x-ray revealed the possibility of bronchiectasis which led to an urgent referral to a lung specialist.

He showed me the grey mottled x-ray and through the fog of my fever I heard him mention my lymph glands again and again. I finally summoned the courage to ask him outright if he thought I might have lung cancer?

"It's hard to prove otherwise without a CT scan" he replied.

Within an hour I had been scanned and was back in his office being shown the 'ground glass' opacity that had been exposed by the scan. Viral and bacterial pneumonia had spread to both of my lungs. I was neutropenic and required immediate admission to hospital.

There was no chance to go home and no opportunity to give my kids one last cuddle when they got home from school. I was too ill to argue and gratefully accepted the hospital bed, the oxygen and drips, wondering to myself whether my wishes for an end to my life were being answered.

I looked up at one stage to see my brother sitting next me.

"What are you doing here?" I asked the guy who usually only travelled to see me on family get togethers.

"I thought I should come and see you in case you died" was his response.

Die? Wasn't that what I had been wishing for these last few months? Was this it? Had the universe delivered what I had been asking for?

Laying there I felt strangely peaceful. The constant chatter in my mind had stopped. The high fever had given way to a lucidness I hadn't experienced before. In what I now know to be a transcendental experience, I felt deeply connected to my inner being.

Stillness at last.

I felt okay. Okay with being with myself. Okay with me.

It was then, in the stillness I realised that I still wanted to live. I wanted to see my children grow up. Laugh with them. Play with them. Love them. I was going to fight this and get home to them.

Later, after leaving hospital and making a full recovery with minimal long term damage to my lungs, I felt lucky to be alive. Every day since that day I wake up grateful to be here.

I retrained as a health and performance coach and functional nutritionist. I read hundreds of books and scientific papers in a bid to learn how to optimise every aspect of my mental and physical health. I sought out the world's best mentors and teachers so I could discover how to combine high performance with optimised health.

I rebuilt my body, mind and spirit using a combination of ancestral wisdom, modern science and biohacks so as to optimise every aspect of my physical and mental being.

I started working with high achieving clients to help them optimize their health and energy and make a bigger impact in the world. In 2018 I felt lucky to meet my friend and mentor, Paul O'Mahony who showed me how to get my message out to the world on a grand scale so that I could reach a wider audience and fulfil my mission of transforming the lives of a million people.

This book is the result of that journey.

I want to thank you for picking it up and for being a part of my mission. I hope that it will impact your health and that of your family and friends in a positive way. This book is your toolkit to help you live younger for longer.

Here's to improving your healthspan and your lifespan so that you can be the best version of you, and live an extraordinary life.

INTRODUCTION

It's time to rethink health.

"You're in pretty good shape for the shape you are in"
- Dr Seuss

Two hundred years ago, modern medicine (medicine as we now know it) started to emerge after the Industrial Revolution. During this time there was rapid growth in economic activity in Western Europe and the Americas. More and more people moved to live in cities which encouraged the spread of diseases such as typhus and cholera. Louis Pasteur pioneered germ theory and created the first vaccine. It wasn't long before vaccines, drugs and surgery were the common mechanisms for treating and slowing the progression of disease.

The 20th century saw dramatic improvements in life expectancy which built upon improvements made in the 19th century. Public health measures contributed to this increase including childhood vaccinations, the introduction of universal health care, medical advances, improved treatment of chronic diseases such as heart disease and cancer as well as societal lifestyle changes including a decline in rates of smoking.

By 2018 life expectancy at birth in England had increased to 79.6 years for males and 83.2 years for females.

It all sounds so positive until you look at the health of these longer-living populations.

In 2015-17, although an English male could expect to live 79.6 years his average ***healthy life expectancy***[1] was only 63.4 years. This means that he would spend 16.2 of those years (or 20 percent) without enjoying good health.

---

1 Healthy life expectancy is an estimate of the number of years lived in 'very good' or 'good' general health, based on how individuals perceive their general health

On average, females live 3.5 years longer than males but even more of that time is spent in poor health. Females experience only 0.4 more years of good health than men. In 2015–17 an English female could expect to live 83.1 years. Twenty three per cent or 19.4 years would expect to be spent suffering health described as 'not good'.

I include these figures not to scare you, ***but to serve as a wake-up call.***

If you want to live life to the full, living not just a long life but a healthy life, you need to be proactive about your health. Not smoking is still one of the most important things you can do to increase your life expectancy. But health is about so much more than this.

What is health?

The Oxford English Dictionary defines health as "the state of being free from illness and injury." This definition considers health from a negative standpoint.

The World Health Organisation (WHO) defines health as "a state of complete physical, mental and social well-being and not merely the absence of disease or infirmity".

My own definition of health is "a state of complete mental, physical, spiritual and social wellbeing".

Being healthy is about unlocking the best version of you.

My goal in writing this book is to help you achieve that state of complete physical, mental, spiritual and social well-being. This book will help you lay the foundations for becoming the most optimised version of you so that you can ***be more, give more, experience more and make a dent*** during the short time you spend on this planet.

Most people are not living life as their best self or living their best life.

Many people are held back by their health in one way or another. Whether that's through brain fog, lowered energy, back pain, excess weight or a chronic health condition such as diabetes or heart disease, their health limits their life.

Consider some examples. You may think that excess tiredness is down to the demands of the project you've just completed or the new addition to your family if you've recently had kids. Your jeans feel a little tighter and the same foods you've always eaten now lead to a little weight gain. Your concentration gives way to scattered thinking and it becomes harder to focus your attention and creativity. Getting into the flow seems ever more elusive. Somehow your joints ache a little bit and your monthly chiropractic visit ceases to alleviate the mild back pain that nags at you.

As time goes on you realise that you're living life at a level of 6 out of 10 as a result of these combined effects.

I wrote this book to teach you how your health might be holding you back from living life at a level of 10 out of 10.

I want to show you how optimising your health is at the foundation of success and longevity in business and in life. My goal is to give you the simple systems, tools and biohacks that will allow you to become the CEO of your health so that you live younger for longer.

Why i wrote this book

As you read in the Preface, in May 2014 after a five year battle with clinical depression, the deterioration in my mental health gave way to a serious decline in my physical health. This wasn't my first experience of ill-health.

In my late 20s I was diagnosed with insulin resistance, Polycystic Ovary Syndrome (PCOS) and Endometriosis. I underwent extensive surgery and was prescribed the diabetic drug Metformin[2]. With a family history of diabetes and heart disease it looked as though I was destined for the same future.

But as you will learn in this book, our genes do not solely determine our destiny.

I have not gone on to develop diabetes and I managed to completely control my blood sugar and put my PCOS into remission with nutritional interventions. I've gone on to have three beautiful children despite being told by multiple doctors that this might not be possible.

There is no 'one-size fits all' approach to health. Everyone is different and unique in their own individual way. We all have different genes, goals, lifestyles and environments in which we exist. Our lives are constantly changing. The perfect diet or fitness plan for you today is unlikely to be the same one that will be right for you in ten years' time. It's also unlikely to be the same one that is exactly right for your partner or friend.

The science of health is constantly changing and evolving. What we assume today may be disproven in the future. As I write this book we are in the middle of a global health pandemic with Covid-19. Many of the world's population are in some form of lockdown

2 Interestingly, metformin is a drug now taken by many biohackers with a view to enhancing longevity.

and what seems true is that we will emerge from this crisis to a different world than we have been used to. No-one could have predicted this. What Covid-19 has highlighted more than ever before is that our health is of paramount importance and we need to be proactive about it.

'Common' is not 'normal'

While many of the chronic diseases we see across the modern world such as heart disease, diabetes and cancer are so common that everyone has experienced or knows someone with one of these, there is a difference between what is 'common' and what is 'normal'.

There are pockets across the world known as the 'Blue Zones' which have the highest concentration of centenarians and supercentenarians - people who live to, or beyond their 110th birthday). There are many people that aspire to living beyond 140 years of age - Dave Asprey, founder of Bulletproofhas spent over $1 million dollars on biohacking with the aim of reaching 180. As Asprey shared with me in an interview on my podcast, High Performance Health, and as he has also shared with FOX Business "by removing risk and by doing the right things with food, exercise and lifestyle I can easily do 120 and the other 50% on top of that comes from something called technology."[3]

Dr David Sinclair, a professor in the Department of Genetics and co-director of the Paul F. Glenn Center for the Biology of Aging at Harvard Medical School says that "Aging is a disease, and that disease is treatable".

While the concept of living forever seems alien or even undesirable to many people, most people desire longevity. Longevity means improving not just your lifespan but your healthspan. No-one wants to live for a long time crippled with disease. But what if you could live for a long time and remain healthy?

What if you could find a way to live younger, for longer?

To have the same energy, mental acuity and physical capacity of a 25 year old, but with all of the experience you have today.

3 https://www.foxbusiness.com/features/this-entrepreneur-claims-he-will-live-to-180

That is the goal of most of my clients and is recognised as what's needed in order to become the CEO of their health.

This book will show you how you can do that too.

According to history books, the oldest living person to date was Jeanne Calment of France who died in 1997 at the age of 122 years. If you live to 100 your chances of living to 110 and becoming a supercentenarian are 1 in a 1000 or 0.001%.

As of 2019 the top ten causes of death in the United States were:

- Heart disease
- Cancer
- Accidents (unintentional injuries)
- Chronic Lower Respiratory Diseases
- Stroke
- Alzheimer's Disease
- Diabetes
- Influenza and Pneumonia
- Kidney Disease
- Suicide

Research indicates that centenarians have postponed, and in some cases escaped major diseases. They are also mostly within a healthy weight range.[4]

As we get older our chances of developing one of the major diseases increases. Many people are unsure of how much control they have over this and believe that genetics play a large part. While the science of aging and chronic diseases is still emerging, one thing seems clear; our genes are not responsible for our destiny. We have greater control over our health outcomes than we first thought. What unites us as a

4 https://www.ncbi.nlm.nih.gov/pmc/articles/PMC5107392/

human race is that we all seem to go after one or more of the same three goals:

- health
- wealth
- happiness.

Just as there are rules for acquiring and maintaining wealth, there are rules that govern the health of our bodies and minds. Many young people feel invincible in their 20s and the concept of growing old feels a long way off, almost as if it's something that happens to 'other people'. As we progress through life, we become more and more aware of our own mortality and the possibility of developing one of the major diseases that limit our lifespan and more significantly, our healthspan. By the time we reach our 40s we all know at least one person who is battling cancer, heart disease or diabetes, whether it's a friend, a relative or even ourselves.

Lots of people don't give this a great deal of thought until it happens to them, but these diseases are not like viruses that we catch and which immediately make us sick. Often they are the result of years of accumulated long-term stress, inflammation or other damage which could have been limited in their extent with the right lifestyle strategies.

For most of my 20s and early 30s, apart from exercising a few times a week and trying to eat healthily I pretty much ignored my health. As a typical "Type A" personality I was focused on driving my career forward and achieving high levels of success and performance. I was relentless in pursuing my goal of partnership at a large corporate law firm. I paid very little attention to circadian alignment, sleep or mental health. It wasn't until I experienced burnout and the slow deterioration of my body and mind, finally culminating in a respiratory infection so severe that it almost took my life, that I realised it was time to change my habits and lifestyle.

My hope is that in reading this book you will apply the principles that I advocate, so that you can optimise every aspect of your body, mind and spirit.

Can I promise you that it will bulletproof you against the major diseases we so commonly see? No, I cannot. What I can guarantee is that it will help to dramatically reduce your risk so that you can improve not just your lifespan but your healthspan. For some this will mean cross-country skiing into their 80s or bringing the right energy to manifest success in their business. For others it will mean being able to run around with their children and grandchildren. For everyone, it will involve looking and feeling younger. For the "Type A" personalities among us, it will bring all of those things and a whole lot more besides!

What this book will give you is a toolkit to help you become healthier, more energized and stronger in body and mind.

This book is written for individuals like yourself who want to know more, be more and achieve more.

My goal in writing this book is not just to help you protect yourself against many of the chronic diseases we see, but to help you optimise the health of your body and mind in a way that enables you to become a better human and to achieve ever-greater levels of success in business, family and life.

As this book will show you, I believe the secret to longevity in business and life is total health optimization. As Robin Sharma, global leadership expert writes in his book ***'The 5am Club, Own Your Morning. Elevate Your Life'***, "one of the keys to legendary, is longevity".

> Use this book as a foundation for health and as a stimulus to do your own research. Take the principles and apply them to your life - the application is key. This book is not designed to be read merely to build your knowledge of health and longevity.

Instead it is designed to be used practically to transform your body, mind and lifestyle. A high-performance mind, body and lifestyle gives you the foundation to achieve your wildest dreams whether that is:

- Succeeding in business and attracting extraordinary levels of wealth
- Having an enduring intimate relationship with your partner
- Being the best parent to your child(ren)
- Having a solid foundation to complete feats of physical and mental endurance
- Manifesting your ideal life.

It's time to rethink health.

Optimal physical and mental health is the very foundation of sustained high performance. It's the unlocking of the best version of you so that you can ***be more, give more, have more and make an impact*** on the world.

Human optimization is where your mind and body **do** exactly **what** you want them to do **when** you want them to do it. Whether that's achieving some feat of physical endurance, bringing the right energy to your family or company, getting into a flow state when you need to, or improving your clarity and decision making, this book will give you the practical tools to do that.

The life you are experiencing today is the accumulated result of the decisions that you have made to this point. I want to help you to make the right decisions so that you can experience high levels of energy, health and happiness and live an extraordinary life.

I want to help you live younger for longer.

Chapter 1
THE MOST OPTIMISED VERSION OF YOU

"Beauty begins the moment you decide to be yourself"
Coco Chanel

"Welcome" says the server, handing you a glass of bubbly as you walk into the room. You take a quick glance around searching for anyone you know so that you can join their conversation. As you quickly scan the space your eye catches one person across the room. They are standing at the centre of a small group of people who are listening intently, gently nodding their heads and occasionally laughing. It's clear that each member of that group is captivated by the speaker and have been drawn to them, as are you. You find yourself struck by their radiance and energy. Like a favourite song, they seem to be inviting you to dance.

You find yourself walking towards them until you're around half way there when a voice in your head asks where you're going. You don't even know this person. Yet, there seems to be a gentle, alluring pull that magnetically draws you closer to them. You're close enough now to get a good view and you pause for a moment, simply observing.

This person stands tall with their shoulders back, epitomising a calm confidence. But that's not it - you've encountered confident people before. This time it's different. It's not the air of confidence about this person that draws you towards them, but rather it's their aura. They exude a magnetic energy. You can't pin it down to one thing. Could it be their radiant glowing skin? The twinkle in their eye? Their strong, lean body? Their captivating smile? Their eloquent conversation?

Or is it the intoxicating blend of everything together?

You look around the room and notice the beautiful woman in the black dress with her glowing skin; the successful businessman who roars loudly, his waistline testament to the overindulgence that a rich life has enabled; the muscular fit young man in the centre who captivates the attention of beautiful women; the funny man with the glasses that has his group hysterically laughing.

You realise that these people all have their individual attributes - we are all talented in one way or another. And then you look back at the person you first set your eyes on and you realise the difference.

This person has it all together. They leave you in no doubt that they can be, do or have anything they want. From generating extraordinary levels of wealth, to competing in fitness events, running around and playing with their children or grandchildren, this person has it all.

They seem to be in complete control of themselves, in command of their life. They are able to use their mind to tap into unlimited levels of creativity, focus and brilliance whenever they want to. They wake up each morning refreshed, recharged and ready to seize the day. They live life in the moment, bringing total presence to each situation they are in. Their body is lean, strong and flexible.

Each year that goes by brings them richer experiences from which to draw. Their glowing skin and radiant energy belies the fact that they are getting older. Somehow they have defied the rules of aging, possessing the mind and body of a younger person but with the experiences that match the extraordinary life they've lived.

And then it dawns upon you - ***this person is in control.***

This person is achieving not just longevity, but juvenescence - a state of youthfulness.

You quickly recall the goals you wrote out this morning, the same ones you remind yourself of every morning. They fall into three categories. Abundant health. Abundant wealth. Abundant joy.

Health, wealth and happiness. This person has it all. This person is living the dream.

It hits you like a bolt from the blue. This person is in complete control of their mind, body and spirit. They have mastered the art and science of controlling their biology and physiology so that they can be the best version of themselves.

They are living younger, for longer.

You can do the same. This book will show you how.

It all starts the night before...

Chapter 2
SLEEP - THE UNDERRATED KEY TO HEALTH, BEAUTY, LONGEVITY AND SUCCESS

"Sleep is the greatest legal performance enhancing drug that most people are probably neglecting"
Matthew Walker, Why We Sleep

Why start the book with sleep? The truth is that sleep is your number 1 SUPERPOWER.

As Matthew Walker acknowledges, sleep is the "greatest legal performance enhancer for athletes" and they know it.

When you get enough sleep you feel on fire, you perform better, you have stronger mental focus, greater emotional regulation and resilience, your metabolism functions better, hormones are balanced, cortisol (the stress hormone) is lowered, you have better blood sugar regulation, your skin looks healthier and you glow from the inside out.

It also makes each of the other three pillars of living younger, longer much easier to put in place. You will learn what these are as we progress through the book.

To understand the importance of sleep, consider an example. Let's say that you are looking to lose weight. Being underslept has been shown to affect weight loss directly. In one study a group of men and women were placed on a strict calorie controlled diet in a medical centre for 2 weeks. One half were given 5.5 hours of sleep and the other half, 8.5 hours of sleep. In the group that slept for 5.5 hours, 70% of the pounds lost came from muscle mass, not body fat. In the group that slept for 8.5 hours each night, 50% of the pounds lost came from fat, while preserving muscle. As Matthew Walker writes in his book ***'Why We Sleep'***, when you are not getting enough sleep "the body becomes especially stingy about giving up fat". Poor quality, short-duration sleep may also in and of itself promote obesity and diabetes risk.[5]

Sleep is probably the most overlooked and underrated secret weapon we have. It is also the one fundamental that I neglected for many years of my adult life, surviving instead on caffeine and energy bars before I finally burned out.

I'm not the only one who has made such an error. Over the last 30 years the number of adults that are sleep deprived (getting less than 6 hours of sleep per night) has increased significantly. This has become even more pronounced with the lines between work and home becoming blurred, and digital technology becoming such an integral part of our lives.

More than 50 million Americans suffer from over 80 different sleep disorders. Another 20 to 30 million Americans suffer intermittent sleep problems each year. 25 percent of adults in the US report insufficient sleep at least 15 days out of every month. According to the National Institute of Health it is predicted that by the middle of the 21st century, over 100 million Americans will experience difficulty falling asleep.

The impact of sleep loss is huge. Sleepiness affects alertness, vigilance, hand-eye coordination, reaction times, learning ability, mood and the accuracy of short-term memory. Sleepiness leads to an increase in the number of on-the-job accidents and road traffic accidents. Gallup polls studying sleep during the years from 1990 to 2013 indicated that 40% of Americans get less than seven hours of sleep per night.

So many of us actively delay sleep and put it off. According to the National Sleep Foundation, man is the only mammal to willingly

5 https://www.ncbi.nlm.nih.gov/pubmed/19444258

delay sleep. With so many benefits arising from it, why do we consistently put off sleep?

The highest performing athletes such as Roger Federer, Usain Bolt and Lebron James all prioritise their sleep. Roger Federer claims to sleep for 12 hours per day with 9-10 hours at night and a 2 hour nap during the day. Usain Bolt apparently broke a world record having only woken up around 35 minutes beforehand.

Sleep doesn't just enhance your performance on the day; it's also critical for recovery and lowering chronic inflammation. It speeds up healing and protects against chronic diseases.

THE EFFECTS OF SLEEP DEPRIVATION

After twenty-two hours without sleep, human performance is impaired to the same extent as someone who is legally over the alcohol limit for driving.[6]

6 Matthew Walker, "Why We Sleep"

SLEEP AND CANCER RISK

Lack of sleep has been shown to increase risk of certain types of cancer (see also the section on melatonin below). Dr Michael Irwin of the University of California performed landmark studies to show how quickly short sleep duration can affect cancer-fighting immune cells.

In a study of young men, Dr Irwin found that after one single night of going to bed at 3am and waking up at 7am there was a 70 per cent reduction in circulating Natural Killer Cells relative to an eight hour night of sleep. Night time shift work has also been associated with an increased risk of developing a number of different types of cancer including breast, colon, prostate and uterine cancers. A large European study of close to 25,000 individuals, found that sleeping six hours or less was associated with a 40% increased risk of developing cancer relative to sleeping 7 hours each night or more.

One reason sleep scientist, Matthew Walker gives for this, is the increase in inflammation that is prompted by the body's level of sympathetic nervous system activity. He explains that some cancer cells attract the inflammatory factor into the tumour mass to help initiate the growth of blood vessels that feed it with oxygen and nutrients. These in turn help the tumour to grow. The inflammatory factors may also assist in the spread of the cancer - a state known as metastasis.

SLEEP AND CARDIOVASCULAR RISK

Lack of sleep also has deleterious effects for the cardiovascular system. Each year when 1.6 billion people move to daylight savings time, reducing their sleep by one hour there is an increase of 24% in heart attacks the following day. In the autumn when we gain one hour of sleep we see a 21% reduction in heart attacks. The same profile is indicated for car crashes and suicide rates at these times of year.[7]

7 Matthew Walker TED Talk, April 2019

SLEEP AND WEIGHT GAIN

While not necessarily causative, there seems to be a correlation between less sleep and an increase in obesity. During the 1940s, less than 15% of the US population was obese with individuals achieving an average of 8-9 hours sleep each night. Compare this to the early 21st century when obesity rates in the US had risen 30% and the average night's sleep had dropped to less than 7 hours. Research indicates that as sleep has declined, weight has increased.

Lack of sleep has also been associated with a number of other factors including changes in genetic activity and damage to telomeres (which are the protective caps at the end of your chromosomes). It is also responsible for reduced levels of testosterone in men (five hours of sleep per night for one week ages a man by 10-15 years in terms of testosterone production)[8] and lowers sperm count. It also increases your risk of depression, Alzheimer's disease, hypertension and diabetes.

To start improving your sleep you first need to understand what sleep is, how much you need and what a good night's sleep looks like.

8 Matthew Walker, Why We Sleep

HOW MUCH SLEEP DO YOU NEED?

The amount of sleep that you need varies from person to person, but it is generally accepted that most adults need between 7 to 9 hours of sleep each night. The table below shows the optimal amount of sleep you should be striving to get according to age.[9]

Age	Recommended	May Be Appropriate	Not Recommended
Newborns 0-3 months	14 to 17 hours	11 to 13 hours 18 to 19 hours	Less than 11 hours More than 19 hours
Infants 4-11 months	12 to 15 hours	10 to 11 hours 16 to 18 hours	Less than 10 hours More than 18 hours
Toddlers 1-2 years	11 to 14 hours	9 to 10 hours 15 to 16 hours	Less than 9 hours More than 16 hours
Preschoolers 3-5 years	10 to 13 hours	8 to 9 hours 14 hours	Less than 8 hours More than 14 hours
School-aged Children 6-13 years	9 to 11 hours	7 to 8 hours 12 hours	Less than 7 hours More than 12 hours
Teenagers 14-17 years	8 to 10 hours	7 hours 11 hours	Less than 7 hours More than 11 hours

9 https://www.sleepfoundation.org/press-release/national-sleep-foundation-recommends-new-sleep-times

Young Adults 18-25 years	7 to 9 hours	6 hours 10 to 11 hours	Less than 6 hours More than 11 hours
Adults 26-64 years	7 to 9 hours	6 hours 10 hours	Less than 6 hours More than 10 hours
Older Adults ≥ 65 years	7 to 8 hours	5 to 6 hours 9 hours	Less than 5 hours More than 9 hours

These are only guidelines however, and many factors play a part in the amount of sleep needed including your underlying genetics and the amount of physical activity that you engage in. Many Olympic athletes and professional sportspeople express a need for 10 to 12 hours of sleep in any 24-hour period. As you will see from the table above, more sleep is not always better. For the average adult, sleeping more than 9 hours per night has also been associated with an increased risk of some chronic diseases and a shorter lifespan.

In an ideal world you would get between 7.5 and 9 hours of sleep each night depending on your unique needs and lifestyle demands. This is not always possible of course as life can get in the way, particularly for those in demanding jobs, individuals who travel a lot and also for professional athletes. Nick Littlehales, author of ***'Sleep: The Myth Of 8 Hours The Power Of Naps And The New Plan To Recharge Your Body And Mind'*** has a unique system for dealing with disrupted or shorter nights of sleep. If you're not able to get a minimum of 7.5 to 9 hours of sleep each night, he encourages you to look at getting a total of 35 cycles per week and not fewer than 30 cycles. Each sleep cycle is around 90 minutes in duration (see further below).

If you have missed out on a good night's sleep you may think that taking a nap will make up for the deficit. While a nap can revive you, current sleep research indicates that a nap will not compensate for the enhancing of the complex functions of the brain that take place at night including memory, learning, emotional regulation, decision-making and complex reasoning. As such, regularly short sleeping at night and relying on daytime naps to compensate should be avoided.

That said, naps can be a solid part of your daily routine and even enhance mental performance and productivity in the afternoon. A slight afternoon dip in energy that many experience is very common and represents a message from your body to reboot. There are a number of techniques that can be used to achieve this reboot (see the later chapter on Stress, Resilience & Recovery) and good nutrition can help to avoid the slump being too profound (see Chapter 4).

Many people are concerned that if they have a nap in the afternoon they will be considered lazy or unproductive. This has not been shown to be the case, however.

A study by the University of California in San Diego demonstrated the performance benefits of an afternoon nap. Subjects were quizzed pre- and post-nap and their brain activity was monitored using an fMRI machine. In contrast to the control group, the nappers' neurons were significantly brighter post-nap and these subjects functioned as well in the afternoon as they did in the morning. The brain activity in the subjects that did not have a nap deteriorated over the course of the day.[10]

Some companies such as Google have even gone so far as to install sleep pods in their offices which play calming music to enable employees to take a nap.

---

10 https://www.ncbi.nlm.nih.gov/pmc/articles/PMC2716730/

THE RIGHT LENGTH OF A NAP

There is a perfect length for a nap which will help you avoid feeling groggy and tired when you wake up, but which is sufficient to revitalise you and give you sustained productivity for the next 3 to 4 hours. As Dr Michael Breus explains in his book 'The Power of When', "Performance enhancement from napping is time sensitive". If you nap for too long or too short a time you may not experience the full benefits that you were hoping for. He explains that for performance benefits and the most time efficiency, a 10-minute nap gives most people the best results. This shorter duration nap allows people to transition back into peak alertness more quickly and ensures that the brain benefits for the rest of the working day.

The critical thing when timing a nap is to make sure that you end the nap before you enter in to slow-wave deep sleep. Waking up from a nap (or even a night of sleep) in slow-wave delta sleep will make you feel foggy and groggy upon waking and it can take at least half an hour to feel alert again. There are two options when planning the length of your nap to sharpen your focus for the remainder of the day:

1. Nap for less than 20 minutes or
2. Nap for 90 minutes (completing a full sleep cycle, cycling through deep sleep, back into light sleep).

If you take the option of napping for less than 20 minutes then I would suggest that you set an alarm to avoid accidentally sleeping for longer. An effective strategy for improving the performance enhancing benefits of a nap is to drink an espresso or black coffee approximately 10 minutes before your nap so that the effects of the caffeine are kicking in as you wake.

For most people, a nap of 20 minutes or less will not affect their ability to sleep well the following evening so long as the nap is taken before 2pm and other good sleep hygiene measures explained later in this chapter are also practiced.

A word of caution however; this may not be the case for those who struggle with insomnia. If you struggle to sleep at night you may be better using another of the recovery techniques featured in Chapter 5 instead of a nap to revitalize yourself for a productive afternoon.

THE STAGES OF SLEEP

The current accepted wisdom is that all adults (barring a small minority) require between 7-9 hours of sleep per night. Few people need less than 7 hours per night. It's not just the duration of sleep that matters, but also the quality of sleep. During sleep, we cycle through 4 main stages (explained further below), all of which are important in terms of function. To operate on our 'A game' and look and feel younger than our years, we need to ideally ensure that we are getting sufficient time in each part of the sleep cycles. Each sleep cycle is around 90 minutes and so seven and a half hours of sleep is around 5 sleep cycles.

Deep sleep occurs mostly in the early part of the night. Getting sufficient deep sleep is crucial to releasing enough human growth hormone (a powerful youth enhancer) and for our body's internal repair systems to work properly. Rapid Eye Movement (REM) sleep is most predominant during the sleep cycles of the last third of the night. This is one reason why you should stick to a regular bedtime (more on this later) as it is important to ensure you get enough deep sleep. If you go to bed later in the night you may miss out on the crucial first sleep cycles of deep sleep and go straight to the REM-dominated cycles. Similarly if sleep is cut short by an alarm, you may miss out on sufficient REM sleep.

Both REM sleep and Non-REM sleep (N1-N3) are equally important. Non-REM occurs earlier in the sleep phase while REM is mostly concentrated later. Non-REM is slow wave sleep (~2Hz) and is like billions of neurons singing in synchronicity while REM sleep is fast (50Hz) and looks more like waking brain activity. Typically REM sleep occupies 20-25 per cent of total sleep or approximately 1.5-2 hours of total sleep per night.

Non-REM Sleep consists of three different stages and N1, N 2 and N3. N1 is the first stage of sleep and is the lightest form of sleep where the person is on the border between sleep and wakefulness. During this stage the brain transitions from beta and gamma brain wave states typical of waking state, with frequencies of 12-30Hz and 25-100Hz, to slower more synchronised alpha waves at a frequency of of 8-13Hz before finally moving to theta waves at a frequency of of 4-7 Hz.

Stage 1 Sleep (N1):

N1 sleep is the transition between wakefulness and sleep. Your muscles relax and your breathing rate starts to slow. During N1 sleep you don't usually dream. As your muscles are still active you may suddenly twitch during short micro-awakenings as you start to fall into a deeper sleep. N1 sleep should ideally form between 2% and 5% of your total sleep.

Stage 2 Sleep (N2):

The next stage is N2 sleep and it is during this stage that your awareness of your surroundings starts to fade. Brain waves get progressively slower and are predominantly theta waves, but with occasional interspersed fast waves. It is during this stage that you experience short bursts of electrical activity (12-14Hz) known as sigma waves which last around half a second each. These 'sleep spindles' help with the transfer of memories from the short-term memory to the long-term memory. During Stage 2 sleep your heart rate slows, body temperature decreases and your muscles relax. This is the easiest stage of sleep to wake from.

N2 sleep should form the bulk of the night with around 45 to 50% of your time spent asleep in N2. N1 and N2 together make up what is classified as light sleep.

Stage 3 Sleep (N3):

Deep sleep, also known as N3 sleep, should form approximately 15 to 20% of total sleep. This slow wave sleep is predominated by

Delta brain waves with a frequency of 0.5-4Hz. During this stage your awareness of surroundings is very limited and resting heart rate, breathing rate, blood pressure and neural activity reach their lowest levels. It is during this stage that you are most likely to dream more than in any other non-REM sleep. During N3, memory consolidation and information processing take place. It is during N3 that you are most likely to experience night terrors, sleepwalking or sleep talking.

During N3 sleep your respiration slows, your blood pressure drops and growth hormone is released. This is also when deep tissue repair takes place. The release of growth hormone helps with muscle tissue and also in repairing the lining of the gut which it is estimated is repaired every 10 days. Growth hormone is only produced in the absence of high insulin levels and so consuming your last meal a minimum of 3 hours before bed is important.

Most deep sleep occurs in the first third of the night and so going to bed too late can compromise the amount of deep sleep you get. As Matthew Walker explains, the shift from Non-REM to REM sleep happens at certain times of the night regardless of when you go to bed. If you go to bed very late at night (e.g. 3am) then your sleep will naturally move towards more REM-heavy sleep, missing out on the deep restorative repair that occurs in slow-wave sleep. This shift to REM dominated sleep will in part be affected by your chronotype with so-called 'night-owls', thought to have a bit more flexibility in the time they are able to go to bed as they naturally wake up later.

During deep sleep you are hard to rouse and if you do wake up, you are likely to feel groggy. Using an alarm such as the one featured on the app, 'Sleep Cycle' can be helpful in avoiding waking up during deep sleep as these alarms contain features that wake you when you are in lighter sleep. If you do wake up during deep sleep it can take at least 30 minutes to shake off the groggy feeling and to feel mentally alert. This is one of the main reasons that napping for longer than 20 minutes but less than 90 minutes can lead to you waking up feeling particularly groggy and lethargic.

Rapid Eye Movement (REM) Sleep:

REM sleep is a lighter form of sleep than Stage 3 sleep and is the time during which your eyes move back and forth. During this stage your blood pressure, heart rate and body temperature all rise. Your muscles are paralyzed since this is the time during which you are most likely to dream and without the paralysis of muscles, you would act out your dreams. Brain waves are faster during REM sleep and similar in length to brain waves during wakefulness. Most REM sleep occurs during the final third of the night. It makes up between 20-25 percent of our sleep.

All stages of sleep are very important. No aspect of our biology is left unscathed by sleep deprivation; as Matthew Walker says "It sinks down into every possible nook and cranny..."

What Happens During REM And Non-REM Sleep?

REM sleep is responsible for forming new neural connections, dreaming, problem solving, empathy and blunting emotional responses to painful memories. You may have heard the expression that time is a great healer but as sleep scientist, Matthew Walker explains, it's the time spent during REM sleep that provides emotional convalescence, lowers anxiety and regulates cardiovascular function. REM sleep helps us to cement our memories. During REM sleep there is activation of the cardiovascular system with high activation and then a fall in activation. REM Sleep affects heart rate variability - an indicator of how well the sympathetic and parasympathetic branches of the nervous system communicate with each other.

Non-REM is responsible for pruning memories, transferring short-term memory to long-term memory (especially important if you are trying to learn something), gaining 'muscle-memory', the release of growth hormone and parasympathetic nervous system activation. Slow wave, deep sleep enables a homeostatic recalibration of blood pressure and lowers systemic blood pressure in the morning relative to the evening. Aging has been shown to reduce slow-wave deep sleep with faster frequency brain wave activity which seems to correlate with poor cardiovascular outcomes. Deep sleep resets cardiovascular tone.

Consumption of alcohol close to bedtime can reduce the amount of REM sleep and is one of the key reasons that individuals who have consumed significant amounts of alcohol may not remember what happened the night before. Their memories are simply not formed. One study showed that students who consumed any alcohol remembered less than those who did not.

Ideally, REM sleep should form 20-25% of total sleep with approximately 20% being deep sleep. Deep sleep seems to decline with age and so ensuring that you are doing the right things to get enough deep sleep is key, particularly as you get older.

How can you ensure that your sleep architecture is as good as it can be so that you wake up feeling refreshed and revitalised?

Setting a constant wake up time is one of the most powerful tools to enhance recovery - says Nick Littlehales, author of 'Sleep' and advisor to elite athletes and football teams.

Choose your earliest wake up time and then count back 5 sleep cycles from your wake up time. So for 7.5 hours if you need to be up by 6am, then you need to be in bed asleep by 10.30pm.

There is a very tiny percentage of the population that needs five hours sleep or less per night. In fact, there is a gene (a subvariant of BHLHE41) that is deemed to be so rare that according to Dr Thomas Roth at the Henry Ford Hospital in Detroit, the number of people who can survive on five hours of sleep or less without any impairment, expressed as a percentage of the population and rounded to the nearest whole number is zero.

You are more likely to be struck down by lightning than to possess this gene variant.

ALIGN WITH YOUR SLEEP CHRONOTYPE

Are you someone who struggles to fall asleep early? Do you instinctively hit the snooze button upon waking?

If so, then you may be a night owl. Our inherent sleep chronotype is largely genetic, which you can find out by testing your DNA.

Dr Michael Breus, "America's sleep doctor' has developed a series of questionnaires to determine which of four chronotypes you fall into:

- Bears
- Lions
- Wolves
- Dolphins

According to Dr Breus, bears make up around 50% of the population. They tend to be able to go with the flow, are good sleepers and have a high sleep drive. They have the closest alignment to social norms and the 9-5 routine.

Lions are the early risers. Dr Breus categorises these individuals as the morning-oriented optimists who have a medium sleep drive. They make up around 15-20% of the population. Wolves are equivalent to night owls, the individuals that want to party until the early hours of the morning. They tend to be night-oriented, creative extroverts with a medium sleep drive. Like lions, wolves make up around 15-20% of the population.

Lastly, there are the dolphins. These individuals make up a small subset of the population (around 10%) and are those who are most likely to struggle to sleep. Dr Breus explains that these individuals sleep with half their brain - the other half remains awake and alert. They are the insomniacs with a low sleep drive.

Our sleep chronotype does indeed seem to be largely genetic and you can test your DNA with a simple saliva test to find out your sleep chronotype and better understand your unique circadian rhythm. For more information on testing your DNA, visit www.rethinkhealth.club.

CIRCADIAN RHYTHM

Circadian rhythms are mental, physical and behavioural changes that follow a daily cycle. They are primarily the responses to light and darkness in a person's environment - the instinct to be awake during the day and to sleep at night. The study of circadian rhythms is called chronobiology. Most living things have a circadian rhythm including animals and plants.

BIOLOGICAL CLOCKS

Biological clocks are found in nearly every tissue and organ in the body. They are your innate timing device and consist of specific molecules (proteins) that interact in cells throughout the body.

Biological clocks produce circadian rhythms and regulate timing. Humans and all vertebrates have one master clock called the suprachiasmatic nucleus (SCN) that keeps everything in sync. The SCN is a group of approximately 20,000 nerve cells and is located in the hypothalamus in the brain. It receives direct input from the eyes and responds to light.

The circadian rhythms within the body are affected by internal and external factors. The environment has a big influence upon us with the main cue influencing circadian rhythm being light. Light-dark cycles can be used to speed up, slow down or reset biological clocks and circadian rhythms.

Circadian rhythms influence a multitude of factors in your health, including:

- body temperature
- eating habits
- digestion
- sleep-wake cycles

Biological clocks that run fast or slow can result in disrupted or abnormal circadian rhythms. Irregular circadian rhythms have been linked to a number of chronic health conditions, including:

- sleep disorders,
- obesity,
- diabetes, and
- mood disorders.

The World Health Organisation has categorised night shift work as a probable carcinogen. Managing your exposure to light may be one of the most important things that you can do to enhance your sleep and your overall health.

Assuming that you are not someone who works shifts, the more in tune you can be with your circadian rhythm, the better your sleep will be. It is widely accepted that our 24 hour circadian rhythm is as follows:

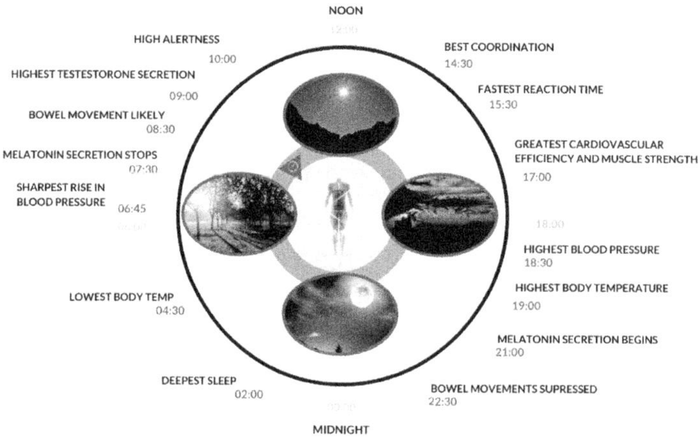

As you will see, melatonin production stops at around 7.30am in the morning. This is preceded by a sharp rise in blood pressure at around 6.45am and a rise in cortisol. Known as the cortisol awakening response (CAR), this is the rise in cortisol concentration that occurs in the first hour after waking from sleep. It is there to get you out of bed and to get going.

Cortisol and melatonin have an inverse relationship with each one only being produced in the right concentrations in the absence of the other.

If you are unduly stressed and do not take the time to wind down properly before bed or if you expose yourself to too much artificial blue light in the evening before bed, insufficient amounts of melatonin will be produced which can lead to you finding it difficult to fall asleep or indeed to stay asleep (see the section on blue light below for further detail).

THE ANTIOXIDANT POWER OF MELATONIN

Melatonin has been shown to have anti-cancer benefits relating to various types of cancers, in particular upon breast cancer cells. In breast cancer, melatonin has been shown to have an effect in disrupting oestrogen-mediated cellular pathways with a reduction in oestrogenic stimulation of cells.[11] A number of studies have shown that a disruption in circadian rhythm, specifically due to night shift work is correlated with an increased risk of developing breast cancer.

One well-established risk factor for breast cancer development is exposure to excessively high levels of estrogen. Some researchers hypothesize that the increased risk of cancer in night shift workers is as a result of an increase in estrogenic activity due to the disruption of melatonin production. Several studies have demonstrated an inverse correlation between melatonin metabolites and a risk of developing breast cancer.

Observational studies show lower levels of melatonin in women with an established diagnosis of breast cancer.

Studies in rodents have confirmed that removal of the pineal gland and/or disruption in circadian rhythm can lead to spontaneous tumor development and increased growth of existing tumours. There is also epidemiological evidence of higher cancer rates in night shift workers. The World Health Organisation's International Agency for Research on Cancer deems that night shift work is "probably carcinogenic to humans (Group 2A)". Based on a 2008 study of 147 communities in Israel it was estimated that light at

11 https://www.naturalmedicinejournal.com/journal/2010-02/overview-melatonin-and-breast-cancer

night (LAN) led to a 73% higher breast cancer incidence compared to the lowest LAN exposed communities.[12]

While studies in rodents that have been pinealectomized and individuals exposed to LAN suggest a causal role between the growth and development of tumours, this is not the only factor at play. The biological effects of exposure to light and dark on the SCN go beyond melatonin production. The light/dark cycle also regulates clock genes which control cell cycle regulatory genes and genes involved in apoptosis (normal cell death).[13] The clock genes act independently of melatonin.[14]

Melatonin is produced from the amino acid L-tryptophan in the pineal gland and also the gastrointestinal tract and lymphocytes.

Melatonin that is produced in the pineal gland is under the control of the SCN and is regulated by the light/dark cycle. The pineal production of melatonin follows a daily rhythm with most of melatonin production beginning after 9pm and peaking at about 2am.

The production of melatonin is triggered by darkness and is suppressed by light. Melatonin that is produced in the pineal gland is under the control of the SCN and is regulated by the light/dark cycle. The brain receives light and dark signals through the retina of the eye. These are then communicated to the SCN, the brain's master bio clock via the optic nerve.

When it is dark the SCN signals the pineal gland to increase production of melatonin. Typically the pineal production of melatonin follows a daily rhythm with most melatonin production beginning after 9pm and peaking at about 2am.

---

12 https://www.ncbi.nlm.nih.gov/pubmed/18293150
13 https://www.ncbi.nlm.nih.gov/pmc/articles/PMC1964886/
14 Stevens RG. Working against our endogenous circadian clock: Breast cancer and electric lighting in the modern world. Mutat Res. 2009;680:106-108, https://www.ncbi.nlm.nih.gov/pubmed/20336819

Melatonin stays low during daylight hours as other hormones rise to help us stay focussed, alert and energised throughout the day.

If you are exposing your eyes to blue light during the course of the evening you are likely to be reducing the production of melatonin which may limit your ability to fall asleep and stay asleep.

Melatonin is not in itself, a sedative. It helps to promote sleep by regulating the body's circadian clock and sleep-wake cycles.

One of the key things you can do to improve your sleep is keep a regular sleep routine, going to bed and waking up at the same time each day, even on weekends (or within 30-60 minutes of your usual sleep/wake time). This helps to improve your sleep-wake cycles. Taking melatonin has also been shown in scientific research that it may help to strengthen and improve sleep-wake cycles and assist in keeping a regular schedule. Research[15] indicates that taking melatonin may shorten the time it takes to fall asleep ('sleep latency'), increase REM sleep[16] and increase the amount of sleep overall.

15 https://www.ncbi.nlm.nih.gov/pubmed/9236698?dopt=Abstract
16 https://www.ncbi.nlm.nih.gov/pubmed/14715839?dopt=Abstract

MELATONIN AS AN ANTIOXIDANT

Melatonin is also a powerful antioxidant and plays an important role in protecting the brain against neurodegenerative diseases and cognitive impairment. Oxidative stress is believed to be one of the key factors in age-related cognitive decline and neurodegenerative diseases such as Alzheimer's disease. As an antioxidant, melatonin may help to protect against cell damage not only in the brain, but also in the cardiovascular system and other physiological systems of the body. According to research, melatonin may also help in lowering high blood pressure.

HOW TO NATURALLY INCREASE PRODUCTION OF MELATONIN

As mentioned above, the correct regulation of light is key to melatonin production with increased melatonin production during darkness. Light at night attenuates melatonin production.

However, there are also important nutrients involved in the production of melatonin. Ensuring that you are getting enough of the right types of foods in your diet can also help to enhance your sleep at night. Folate, zinc and magnesium deficiencies have been linked with lower melatonin levels in rodents and in one study, Vitamin B6 was also shown to be important in increasing melatonin production.[17]

Natural sources of folate, zinc, magnesium and B6 are shown in the table below:

Vitamin/Mineral	Food Sources
Vitamin B6	Asparagus, Bananas, Broccoli, Brussels sprouts, Cabbage, Cauliflower, Eggs, Lentils, Onions, Peppers, Red kidney beans, Salmon, Squash, Tuna, Turkey, Watercress, Wheatgerm
Folate (Vitamin B9)	Asparagus, Avocados, Beans, Broccoli, Cashew nuts, Cauliflower, Chickpeas, Collard Greens, Green Vegetables, Hazelnuts, Kale, Lentils, Mustard Greens, Peanuts, Peas, Romaine Lettuce, Sesame seeds, Spinach, Sprouts, Squash, Turnip Greens, Walnuts, Wheat germ
Magnesium	Avocados, Beans, Dark Leafy Greens, Fish, Nuts, Seeds, Whole Grains
Zinc	Almonds, Beans, Beef, Chicken, Chickpeas, Crab, Lobster, Oysters, Peas

Consuming enough protein is also key to ensuring that you are

17 https://www.ncbi.nlm.nih.gov/pmc/articles/PMC3402070/

getting a good night's sleep. Tryptophan, an essential amino acid (meaning it needs to be obtained from your diet) is necessary for your body to produce serotonin which gets converted into melatonin.

Consuming carbohydrates alongside protein can help to slightly increase the amount of tryptophan in your brain. This happens because carbohydrates promote the release of insulin. Insulin helps move other amino acids besides tryptophan into muscle fat or tissue. The result is more tryptophan than other amino acids in your blood. This can lead to greater levels of tryptophan crossing the blood-brain barrier into your brain. Once in the brain tryptophan is synthesized into serotonin and provided you have the right cofactors and are not exposing yourself to too much blue light, this should result in melatonin being produced too.

The minimum amount of protein to consume is at least 0.55 g of protein per pound of body weight per day. For individuals who experience sleep problems, this can be increased to up to 0.7 to 0.8 g of protein per pound. Note that these represent the minimum amounts, not necessarily what is optimal. For further information on optimising protein requirements see Chapter 4.

If you are following cyclical caloric restriction, increasing your protein intake throughout the day on lower calorie days may help with enhancing sleep. Supplementing with 10 to 20g of essential amino acids (EEAs) can be a useful strategy for those individuals on a lower calorie intake.

It may also be worth supplementing magnesium in your diet.

Magnesium assists in the conversion of 5HTP to melatonin. The most absorbable forms of magnesium are magnesium citrate, glycinate, taurate and aspartate. Magnesium glycinate can be particularly helpful in aiding relaxation and enhancing sleep. Effective daily doses of magnesium are between 200 and 500mg. Start slow and test your tolerance as higher levels of certain types of magnesium can result in loose bowel movements. According to the World Health Organization as many as 75% of US adults do not meet the US Food and Drug Administration's Recommended Daily Intake of 420 mg of magnesium.

SUPPLEMENTARY MELATONIN

MELATONIN

At the time of writing, melatonin is only available in the UK on prescription. It is readily available in many parts of the USA and can be useful when travelling to adjust to time zones. Board certified sleep specialist, Dr Michael Breus and author of 'The Power of When' says not to use it regularly. It can create a dependency where you need more and more for it to remain effective, or you may inhibit your body's ability to use it effectively. Many people also take unnecessarily high doses of melatonin. A microdose as low as 0.3mg can be effective to improve sleep.

OTHER SUPPLEMENTS TO HELP WITH SLEEP

L-theanine is an amino acid found in green tea leaves and can be taken in supplement form. L-theanine has been shown to increase relaxation and reduce stress. It increases alpha brain waves and helps in falling asleep. [18]Research shows that L-theanine crosses the blood brain barrier in approximately 30 minutes and helps to improve mental relaxation without loss in alertness. It can be consumed alongside caffeine to reduce the jittery effect that some people experience. Once it crosses the blood-brain barrier, L-theanine has been shown to reduce cortisol levels and anxiety. When combined with caffeine, L-theanine has been shown to improve performance on cognitively demanding tasks in a ratio of 1:2 (caffeine: L-theanine). If you consume 100mg of caffeine then you would take 200 mg of L-theanine alongside it. [19]

Vitamin D deficiency has also been implicated in poor sleep quality. Dark skin tone, obesity, limited sunlight exposure and a genetically reduced ability to synthesise vitamin D from sunlight have all been implicated in lower vitamin D levels. You can check your ability to synthesise Vitamin D with a simple DNA test (see chapter resources for details). Vitamin D should be taken with fatty foods to enhance absorption and alongside vitamin K2 to to limit the risk of high blood calcium levels. Vitamin D should not be taken in the evening as this can interfere with melatonin production.

Taurine, a non-essential amino acid (meaning the body can produce it), also found in meat and fish has been shown to decrease stress and anxiety and also to increase the amount of GABA, an anxiety-inhibiting neurotransmitter. Taking 3g of taurine can be helpful in enhancing sleep especially when taken alongside magnesium.

18 https://koreamed.org/SearchBasic.php?RID=0124KJN/2003.36.9.918&DT=1
19 https://www.ncbi.nlm.nih.gov/pubmed/18681988

SOUND AND THE IMPACT ON SLEEP

Sound can have an impact on sleep quality and if you live in a noisy neighbourhood you may need some help blocking out the noise - ear plugs and white/pink noise devices can help with this.

Music can actually be used to enhance deep states of relaxation and improve your quality of sleep. A practice known as brainwave entrainment is the practice of bringing your brain wave frequencies in sync with an externally produced frequency. When you are in deep sleep or deeply relaxed, theta and delta brain waves dominate. You can use a brain entrainment device to move you into theta and delta brain waves. The sound frequencies that are typically used to do this are binaural beats.

Binaural beats are two different tones that are close in frequency and are played together, one in each ear - to get the full benefits, you will need to wear headphones to get the full effect of this. When both sounds enter the brain they combine to a frequency that represents the difference between the original frequencies. Depending on the difference in frequency created, you can induce the brainwave state that you are looking for. The 'Pzizz' app and 'Sleepstream' app both produce relaxing sounds that are combined with binaural beats. The Sleepstream app also allows you to choose settings that can be used to enhance focus and creativity.

THE POWERFUL EFFECTS OF LIGHT ON SLEEP

Bright blue or white light before bed is kryptonite for sleep. New LED and compact fluorescent light bulbs have an intensity of blue light that we have not yet developed as humans to handle. They don't contain the other spectrums of light that are contained in sunlight such as infrared, red and violet light. Recent studies indicate that this 'junk' light is potentially as damaging to our bodies as junk food is. It can cause inflammation and damage to mitochondria.

Blue light can disrupt the quality of your sleep in two main ways:

3. It suppresses melatonin production - which as you learnt earlier is critical to falling asleep, staying asleep and protecting you against certain types of cancer.
4. Blue light stimulates a type of light sensor in your brain known as intrinsically photosensitive retinal ganglion cells (ipRGCs) in the retina. These sensors communicate with the circadian clock telling you when it's time to sleep and wake up.[20]A 2014 study found that people who read from a blue light emitting device at night took longer to fall asleep and had less deep sleep than those subjects who read from a printed book.[21]

Other health issues associated with blue light include an increased risk of developing breast cancer and prostate cancer[22] and macular degeneration[23] (damage to the retina that can lead to vision loss).

---

20 https://www.ncbi.nlm.nih.gov/pubmed/26900325
21 https://www.pnas.org/content/pnas/112/4/1232.full.pdf
22 https://www.ncbi.nlm.nih.gov/pubmed/29687979
23 https://www.ncbi.nlm.nih.gov/pubmed/26900325 **

HOW YOU START YOUR DAY IMPACTS YOUR SLEEP AT NIGHT

How well you sleep at night begins with your activity first thing in the morning. Getting outside and accessing natural sunlight in the early part of the morning can really help to align circadian rhythm. As Ben Greenfield writes in his book 'Boundless', research suggests that 30 minutes of moderate-intensity aerobic exercise at 65% of maximum heart rate prior to breakfast is beneficial for enhancing sleep the following night. Ideal forms of exercise to achieve this would be a walk or yoga. As already mentioned, cortisol is at its highest in the morning and this type of exercise will not raise cortisol unduly highly which can otherwise lead to a big spike in appetite and overeating. Greenfield also advocates longer workouts between 2pm and 6pm at 50 to 80% of VO2max which can improve sleep. Thirty minutes of high intensity exercise at 85 to 90% of maximum heart rate to exhaustion for 30 minutes, 3 to 4 hours before bedtime has been shown to help to decrease sleep latency (the time it takes to fall asleep) and improve sleep efficiency.

Exercise naturally increases the core temperature of the body and the activity of the sympathetic nervous system for a few hours afterwards. If you are exercising close to bedtime, engaging in activities designed to stimulate the parasympathetic nervous system such as meditation or breath work can help to improve sleep quality as can activities that lower the core temperature of the body such as cold showers.

The first hour of your day defines the rest of your day - in terms of mood, productivity, focus and effectiveness. For more tips on how to optimise daily productivity and performance see Chapter 5 .

HOW TO SET YOURSELF UP FOR A GREAT NIGHT OF SLEEP:

1. **WAKE UP AT THE SAME TIME EACH DAY**

   Set an alarm to wake up at the same time each day, even on weekends (or at the very least within 30-60 minutes of your usual wake up time). We are not always able to control the time that we go to sleep, but we can control the time that we wake up on a consistent basis. If you have had a late night, it is still better to start your day at the same time and take a nap in the afternoon rather than mess up your circadian rhythm with a long lay-in, which can have a detrimental effect for much of the following week.

   To avoid being roused from a deep slumber you can time your bedtime by counting back in 90 minute cycles from when you plan to wake up and add around 15 minutes to fall asleep. For example, if you have had friends for dinner and they don't leave until 12.30pm and your usual wake-up time is 6am, then you may wish to go to bed at 1am and wake up slightly later at 7.30am. This would give you 4 cycles instead of the usual five. Waking up at, or within an hour of your usual wake up time doesn't preclude you from a "lazy Sunday morning". You can still lounge in bed, read, make love or anything else you enjoy, just making sure that you are awake. You could then follow this with a nap in the early afternoon to help you get through the rest of the day.

   To make things even simpler you can use an app such as 'Sleep Cycle' which senses when you are in lighter sleep and will wake you within thirty minutes of your designated alarm time. Using a sunrise alarm clock which simulates sunrise can also be a powerful tool.

2. **DO NOT HIT THE SNOOZE BUTTON.**

   This is important for two key reasons.

   Firstly, as Matt Janes, Neuroscientist and Functional Medicine Practitioner explains "When your alarm sounds in the morning, you are torn out of restful sleep. This shock quickly engages your sympathetic nervous system, the fight or flight branch of your autonomic nervous system". Repeatedly hitting the snooze button re-engages the fight or flight response "compounding the negative physiological effects on your body, including the release of cortisol which, when prolonged, can create inflammation on a cellular basis".

   Secondly, hitting the snooze button and delaying getting out of bed is failing to follow through on an earlier commitment you make to yourself from the very first point of the day. When you set your alarm clock before going to sleep, you effectively make a promise to yourself to get up at that time. In hitting the snooze button you are letting yourself down. This is a powerful signal to yourself and can affect your self-esteem and your self-confidence. It is not the best way to frame the day and the way that you start the day sets the tone for the rest of the day.

3. **GET OUTSIDE.**

   Go outside in the early part of the day and access natural sunlight. This is important for aligning your circadian rhythm. Try to spend a minimum of 15-20 minutes outside in the early morning. This can involve drinking your morning cup of tea or coffee outside, doing some yoga or stretching or going for a walk. The main thing is to get outside and expose your skin to the natural daylight.

4. **ENJOY YOUR "POWER HOUR".**

Your first hour of the day should be something that you both look forward to and which sets you up for the day ahead. This will help to ensure that you deliver on your promise of getting out of bed as soon as the alarm goes off. It also helps you ease into your day so that you are starting the day intentionally and with full presence while engaging in activities that will set you up for a purposeful, productive and high performing day ahead. For more tips on optimising your morning routine with powerful daily rituals, see Chapter 5.

5. **BOOKEND YOUR WORK DAY.**

Closing off the end of your working day is a powerful way to transition from work to relaxation time. To continue to perform at high levels and optimise our body and mind we need to build in recovery cycles. Our bodies and minds are not designed to be pushed and pushed until we eventually collapse into bed only to find that we then either can't sleep or wake in the middle of the night thinking about the next day and our never-ending to do list.

Set a 'finish work time' at the start of each day and always aim to finish then or within 30 minutes of that time. This will ensure that you only focus on the highest value tasks and actually work for all the time you work (more on this in Chapter 5). At the end of your day, spend a few minutes journaling on what you achieved, what your number one task is for the next day and what you learnt. These activities will free up mental space and help you to sleep better.

6. **STOP EATING AND DRINKING AT LEAST THREE HOURS BEFORE BED.**

Stop eating and drinking three hours before bed. This will help to keep insulin levels low, lower your resting pulse, lower body temperature and prepare the body for sleep.

7. TAKE A SHOWER OR BATH.

A cold shower or a warm shower/bath can both help to encourage sleep. For some people a cold shower cools the body ready for sleep while for others a warm shower or bath relaxes them especially when combined with magnesium salts and/or essential oils. Experiment with what works for you. Using a natural body cream with essential oils such as lavender can help to encourage better sleep. For suggestions see the chapter resources at www.rethinkhealth.club.

8. DIGITAL SUNSET.

Ninety minutes before bed, stop using electronic devices or watching television, or if this is not possible wear a pair of blue light blocking glasses. These are not all created equal and quality matters and so avoid cheap pairs which do not always block out sufficient amounts of blue light in order to make a material difference. For suggestions see the chapter resources at www.rethinkhealth.club.

9. KEEP THE ROOM COOL.

To sleep well, your core temperature should decrease by 2-3 degrees Fahrenheit (approx 1 degree Celsius). The room temperature should be around 65 degrees Fahrenheit. Being cooler helps to facilitate the naturally timed release of melatonin. Wear minimal clothing and use light bedding (and consider a device such as the Chilipad if struggling to control body temperature). Sleeping with hands and feet out of the covers can help to release excess heat from the body.

10. ENSURE ADEQUATE VENTILATION

Make sure that the room is well ventilated with good quality air. Consider buying an air purifier.

RETHINK > > >

TRADITIONAL THINKING:

- Sleep can be caught up on at weekends and while on vacation.
- High achievers need to sleep less to get ahead and achieve their goals.
- Lack of sleep can be overcome by extra caffeine or energy drinks without adversely affecting our health.

RETHINK:

- A good night's sleep is not optional.
- We can't 'catch up' on sleep.
- Sleep is fundamental to looking, feeling and living younger.
- Sleep helps to protect us against many chronic diseases and renews the health of our mind and body.
- Sleep makes us better and more productive at everything we do.
- Sleep is a performance enhancer.

For more resources on sleep, visit the chapter resources at www.rethinkhealth.club.

Chapter 3
MOVE YOUR BODY

"All truly great thoughts are conceived while walking"
Friedrich Nietzsche

MOVEMENT & EXERCISE

Many people get confused by movement and how much exercise they should be doing each week to stay lean and healthy

If you've got this far in the book I'm going to assume that like me, you want to live a long time and look good while doing it! What many people look for, both men and women, is some muscular definition so that they look good in their clothes and their swimwear. This healthy, athletic look comes from having sufficient muscle mass to give you that definition. Don't worry, what I cover here isn't going to transform you into a muscle-bound bodybuilder! It's what's been scientifically shown to help defy the loss in muscle mass that is associated with aging (known as sarcopenia), protect your bones and give you that lean and athletic look.

In this chapter I am going to cover how much exercise you should be doing each day and each week to increase not just your life span but your health span, and how you can look good while doing it.

GOVERNMENT EXERCISE GUIDELINES

Current government advice in the UK is to exercise at a moderate intensity for 150 minutes each week or at a vigorous intensity for 75 minutes each week.

Like much of the advice that we receive from governments across the world, in my opinion this guidance falls short. The definition of 'moderate intensity' is an activity such as cycling or a brisk walk. If you want to stay lean and healthy and live a long time looking good while doing it, then this falls far short of the amount of exercise you need to take. The average person walks at a speed of 3.1 miles per hour (or 5 km per hour). A brisk walk would be at around 4.5 mph or 7.2 km per hour. Let's assume that you are walking at 4.5 mph and that you do so for 150 minutes per week. This equates to 11.25 miles or 18 km per week. 18 km equates to approximately 23,620 steps. This is approximately 3374 steps each day. For anyone who has tracked their daily steps on a wearable device, you would need to be pretty sedentary to only achieve 3374 steps in a day.

This advice also doesn't take account of the need to use resistance training to avoid sarcopenia. Sarcopenia is the loss of skeletal muscle mass and function which commonly happens with age. During your early thirties you start to lose muscle mass and function. It is estimated that physically inactive people can lose as much as 3 to 5% of their muscle mass each decade after the age of 30.

Simply walking 3374 steps or 2.5 kilometres per day is unlikely to stave off the sarcopenia that occurs as a natural part of ageing.

Let's talk about what you really need to be doing to live a long and healthy life and look good at the same time.

MOVE MORE

My first suggestion is to move more. Many people spend around 8 hours each day sitting through a combination of work, their daily commute and watching television in the evening. The truth is that sitting for this extended period of time is unlikely to counterbalance the amount of food that most people are eating between breakfast, lunch, dinner and snacks and this is regardless of whether they fit in a workout at the beginning or end of the day.

Sitting has been dubbed 'the new smoking', as habitual sedentary behaviour has been associated with an increased risk of type 2 diabetes, obesity, cardiovascular disease, metabolic syndrome and premature mortality. Sitting for long periods of time on a regular basis has been shown to cause changes in glucose transport, insulin signalling and the activity of lipoprotein lipase which is the primary enzyme responsible for breaking down fats. In the same way that you can't outrun a bad diet, you can't outwork a day spent sitting down with an hour spent in the gym. Sitting for extended periods or static standing may also place you at a greater risk of suffering heart issues during exercise. As Ben Greenfield writes in his book ***'Boundless: Upgrade Your Brain, Optimise Your Body And Defy Aging'***, a hard workout at the end of the day of sedentary activity results in an attempt to force blood through 'kinked' vessels". He explains that a formal workout at the beginning or end of the day is not necessary for weight loss. For weight loss, low level physical activity throughout the day is needed.

If you have a desk job you may be wondering how you can achieve this? Here are some easy hacks which are designed to improve your low level endurance and fitness by getting moving throughout the day and improving blood flow. These will help, not just with the health of your body, but also the health of your brain, improving mental focus and acuity.

The first step is to set a timer and get up and move every 15 to 20 minutes. Joan Vernikos, advisor to NASA and author of ***'Sitting Kills, Moving Heals: How Everyday Movement Will Prevent Pain, Illness & Early Death - & Exercise Alone Won't'***, says being sedentary is like going out of your gravitational pull, something that actually ages you. She suggests that you move every 15 to 20 minutes. After 20 minutes of inactivity, she says that your body starts to change in suboptimal ways. Even if all you did was to stand up and shake out your body you would be benefiting it.

For an even better approach, you can install an under-desk treadmill (as I have) so that you can walk while you work. If you are sitting for any length of time, set a timer for every 15 to 20 minutes to stand up and do some stretching or a quick burst of activity. In addition to my under-desk treadmill, I keep a mini-trampoline and a kettlebell in my office and will get up frequently and do any one of the following activities:

- 10 to 15 burpees
- 60 seconds mountain climbers
- 25 jumping jacks
- 15 to 20 kettlebell swings
- 2 minutes of rebounding on the mini-trampoline
- 60 seconds speed rope
- TRX rows.

MOVE IN A FASTED STATE

One of the best things that you can do for fat loss is to exercise in the morning in a fasted state. By that, I don't mean a hard-hitting workout that involves large amounts of muscle glycogen. It is likely that you won't be able to push yourself quite as hard. Secondly, when exercising hard, first thing in the morning you will likely stimulate even greater production of cortisol which is already high in the morning due to the cortisol awakening response which is designed to 'get you going'. Higher levels of cortisol can inhibit fat loss and also lead to fatigue in the mid to late afternoon. Finally a hard hitting early morning workout can lead to overeating later in the day. If this is the only time that you have to exercise on any one given day, then for the most part, a workout is better than no workout. The best time of day to exercise is, after all, the time when you will actually do it!

The type of exercise that I find works best for most people upon waking, which they will actually commit to on a daily basis is some gentle exercise such as a brisk walk or yoga session. You can enhance the fat burning effect of this by consuming a black coffee or green tea before doing this exercise.

You can boost the fat burning effect of this exercise even further by taking a cold shower straight afterwards. If the thought of a cold shower makes you shiver immediately, you can start slowly by simply finishing your usual shower with a 10 to 15 second cold rinse and slowly increase this daily.

WORKOUTS TO ENHANCE LONGEVITY

Now that you have increased your daily movement and are incorporating your morning fasted exercise session into the day, you can begin to add some more structured workouts. For the purposes of looking good and living a long time there are certain types of workouts that you should be hitting each week. These are as follows.

Strength Training / Resistance Training

The first workout that I would suggest is some form of resistance training. As I've already mentioned, we begin to lose lean muscle mass from the age of 30 onwards. As such, you need to fight back against this form of ageing. People often wonder whether they should be doing high repetition, low resistance work or low repetition, high resistance work. This largely depends on your fitness goals and your genetics. Depending on whether you are looking to gain muscle and improve strength or simply burn fat and improve muscle definition, this will play a part in which different rep ranges and levels of resistance that you should focus on. Genetics play a part here and you can easily find out your own unique power, endurance and strength profile through a simple DNA test. For more information on this see the resources at www.rethinkhealth.club.

Bigger muscles are not necessarily better, unless of course that's your thing. What you should be focusing on is maintaining muscle mass while ensuring that the muscle is as strong and functional as possible. This means that you want strong, toned and explosive muscle tissue. The best way to achieve this is to do a number of strength based workouts per week. If you are short on time and you need to keep the number of workouts that you do to a minimum, then you should first focus on scheduling in resistance based workouts.

A very effective and time efficient way to do this is to engage in super slow strength training. The most minimalist way to do this that I have come across was developed by Dr Doug McGuff who co-authored the book, 'Body By Science'. This protocol includes 12 to 20 minutes of what McGuff calls the 'Big Five': extremely slow, controlled lifting of relatively heavy weights. This is intended to increase the time under load (TUL) for muscles which should be between 40 seconds and 150 seconds in total. There is no prescribed number of repetitions for this exercise, instead you should simply be working in a slow and controlled fashion until failure (when you can't perform any more reps with good form). The 'Big 5' exercises are:

- upper Body Push, e.g. machine chest press or bench press,
- upper Body Pull, e.g. seated row or barbell row,
- overhead Push, e.g. overhead press,
- lower Body Push, e.g. squat or leg press, and
- lower Body Pull, e.g. pull down or deadlift.

This workout can be done in less than 12 minutes per week. It's simple and quick. If you want to tweak it slightly to push the muscles even harder, then you can add a burnout set following the initial set where you bang out as many reps as you can at a much lighter weight with speed. You would do this for each of the 5 exercises immediately after doing the super slow set.

While super slow training is very effective, not everyone enjoys this style of training and some people, myself included, prefer a more fluid form of training. By fluid, I mean a style of training that is more continuous and rhythmic in nature, such as performing 3-4 sets of 8-12 repetitions. The most important thing in building muscle and protecting your body against sarcopenia is that you ***progressively overload*** the muscle. This means that you should find it difficult to complete the last 1-2 repetitions of each set with good form.

Another reason that strength training is important is that it can increase your ability to drive glucose into muscle tissue. It has been shown to increase insulin sensitivity and decrease blood glucose levels even if the weights that you are lifting are only 30% of your one rep max (1RM). This is the maximum weight that you can lift for one repetition. Through weight training you will be improving your ability to control your blood sugar and help to reduce the amount of excess sugar that is stored as body fat. This is achieved even with relatively light body weight exercises such as those that form part of the 7-minute bodyweight workout (see below).

HIGH INTENSITY INTERVAL TRAINING

If you are time strapped and need a fast efficient workout that helps you to stave off muscle loss, burn fat and boost metabolism, there are a couple of workouts that have some solid science behind them to help you achieve this.

The 7 Minute Workout

The first is the seven minute workout which was originally published in the American College of Sport Medicine's Health and Fitness Journal. It has been found to have overwhelming health benefits, including weight loss and increased endurance. This is largely due to excess post-exercise oxygen consumption or EPOC. EPOC is the mechanism through which HIIT workouts allow your body to continually burn calories even after you've finished your workout. This is one of the key benefits of HIIT training: maximum results with minimal investment. However, the key thing for this to work is that you must go hard! To benefit from short exercise sessions, you need to work very hard!

Below is the original 'Scientific 7-minute workout' designed by Gretchen Reynolds. The workout is designed to maintain strength and muscle in as little time as possible. Each of the following exercises should be performed for 30 seconds with 10 seconds of rest in between each exercise. Each exercise should be performed as e***xplosively as possible*** trying to achieve as many reps as you can in 30 seconds, except of course for the plank which involves an isometric hold for 30 seconds.

Here are the exercises:

- jumping jacks
- wall sit
- push ups
- abdominal crunch
- step ups
- squat
- tricep dips
- plank
- high knees (running in place)
- lunges (30 seconds each side)
- push-up with rotation
- side plank (30 seconds each side)
-

Tabata Training

The second, even more time efficient (!) style of training is Tabata training. Tabata training was developed by Japanese scientist Dr Izumi Tabata and a team of researchers from the National Institute of Fitness and Sports in Tokyo.

Tabata and his team conducted research on two groups of athletes. The first group engaged in moderate intensity training working out for a total of five days each week for a total of 6 weeks. The second group engaged in high-intensity training, four days each week for a total of 6 weeks. In the high intensity group their workout involved

20 seconds of intense activity with a 10 second rest in between each set for a total exercise time of 4 minutes.

At the end of the 6 week training block both groups had improved their aerobic system (cardiovascular), but the effects were greater in Group 2. Group 1 showed little to no results in their anaerobic system (muscular) whereas Group 2 had improved their anaerobic system by 28 per cent.

What this means is that in just 4 minutes of exercise, 4 times per week, you can enhance both your aerobic and anaerobic systems. Tabata is my 'go to workout' when I have an incredibly busy day and don't have much time for exercise. I also like to do a Tabata set as a break from sitting.

The best exercises to include for a Tabata workout are those that utilise big muscle groups (compound movements). Examples of exercises that you can include in a Tabata workout include pushups, air squats (bodyweight squats), burpees and kettlebell swings.

> You can either pick one and do that same exercise for 8 minutes (harder if you choose an exercise like push ups or burpees - be prepared to get to failure) or mix it up within the sessions. One of my favourite time saving workouts is 2 rounds of Tabata:

- Tabata 1: Air squats
- Tabata 2: Push-ups

*Always remember to warm up first.

High intensity interval training is a very important part of your weekly/biweekly workout routine. Many people push themselves too hard for too long but at the same time, don't push themselves hard enough. What do I mean by this? Some people, particularly weekend warriors and the like, will push themselves for a long period by (for example) going and crushing a triathlon, a long run or a bike ride for 2 to 3 hours, but are not pushing themselves hard enough for a short period of time on a regular basis. By this

I don't mean engaging in a HIIT workout every day as this is likely to raise cortisol, impair recovery and potentially impede your body composition goals. But including some form of HIIT training 1-2 times weekly is both effective and time saving as a means to improving cardiovascular health and where it includes resistance, muscular endurance.

Endurance Training

Overdoing endurance training (extended cardiovascular workouts), may be damaging for your health. In 2012, legendary ultra marathoner Micah True died at the age of 58 years old whilst engaging in a typical easy 12 mile run. This was classed as an easy run because True was used to regularly running 100 miles a day. The results of his autopsy showed that his heart was enlarged and scarred. It is now believed that his death was due to Phidippides cardiomyopathy which is caused by chronic, excessive endurance exercise.

Unless you regularly do long cardio sessions for more than 2 hours at a time, it's unlikely that you need to worry about the Phidippides cardiomyopathy.

Many people mistakenly think that jogging or running melts away body fat and are disappointed when that weight just won't shift or worse they seem to be gaining ever more body fat.

Initially any form of exercise in an untrained individual will pay dividends in the form of fat loss. But over time, why do so many people fail to lose or even gain more body fat with chronic cardio?

The reason for this is that the body will always find the most efficient way to do something. When you are engaging in aerobic exercise on a regular basis such as long cardio sessions with increasing volume and increasing frequency, your body will try to shed any unnecessary excess weight. Unfortunately muscle forms part of this excess weight because it too needs to be carried (it is heavier than fat) and cooled. Body fat on the other hand, is lighter and also provides an almost limitless source of stored usable energy for your body to use for long cardio sessions. This works against your body composition goals not just because you are now storing fat but because having less muscle directly impacts your metabolic rate. The less muscle you have, the less fat you tend to burn because muscle tissue mobilizes stored fat. With the increase in the number and length of aerobic training sessions, your body will become more and more efficient and will start to use less and less of your stored body fat. The times when focusing on cardio sessions to burn fat may be a good idea, are for those overweight individuals who are new to exercise.

For individuals who are already active the best method to burn fat is short high intensity interval cardio sessions. By short, I mean high-intensity sessions that last 30-minutes or less.

In one study, it was found that after 20 weeks of training, participants who performed high intensity interval training lost more body fat than the group who engaged in steady-state endurance training. To avoid falling foul of the SAID principle (which stands for specific adaptation to imposed demands) you should mix up your style of training frequently. The SAID principle states that your body will eventually adapt to the demands that you place upon it. As such, whether that's a regular morning run or a bodyweight HIIT session, you need to mix things up as often as possible. You can do this by swapping between different types of cardio sessions such as rotating between running, cycling, swimming and even trampolining.

You may also mix things up between body weight, resistance training and strength training at high intensity. This may include kettlebell training or moving between dumbbells and barbell training. Adding in full body movements can be particularly effective, for example combining squats with overhead presses, or lunges with bicep curls as this places greater demands on your body. Moving between an upper body exercise and a lower body or full body exercise is also more metabolically demanding, as is using active recovery between sets of resistance training at high intensity.

Examples of such activities include:

- performing a chest press and immediately following it with 20 reps of decline press ups or 60 seconds of body weight squats;
- performing a deadlift clean and press and immediately following it with 30-60 seconds of sprinting.

These kinds of exercises will keep your metabolism 'revs' high and make the workout both more metabolically demanding and time-efficient.

Another way of mixing things up is to perform your workout at a completely different time of day. For example, if you are more of a morning workout person, then doing your workout in the late afternoon can switch things up. The only time that I wouldn't suggest doing this is if you're somebody that struggles with sleep or insomnia, as those individuals benefit from a more regular schedule that is timed with their chronobiology (go back to Chapter 2 on Sleep for more on circadian alignment).

Mixing things up does not mean that you shouldn't have structure to your training regimen. Unless you are new to exercise or in a maintenance phase, constantly switching between modes of exercise and styles of training is unlikely to yield results. Just as the expression "if you want to be a writer, write" holds true, if you want to be a competitive swimmer, you need to swim - a lot! To get good at something or achieve a very specific goal, you need to include specific training to achieve that - 80% of your training should be designed around that goal. For example if you are looking to gain muscle then you need to focus on workouts that help you to build muscle. Alternating cycling with swimming, running, playing sport and the odd strength training workout won't cut it. You need to include 2-5 resistance workouts per week with a small amount of cardio such as a couple of HIIT workouts or LISS (low intensity steady state cardio) workouts thrown in.

With exercise the most important thing to ask yourself is why you are exercising and what you want to achieve and to then design, or work with a professional coach to design your workouts around your goal. For most people, working with a trainer also means that they will work harder as very few people push themselves as hard on their own!

MITOCHONDRIAL TRAINING

Mitochondria are the power sources of your cells. The main currency of energy used by the body is adenosine triphosphate (ATP) and this is created in the mitochondria. Without sufficient mitochondria you will likely feel low on energy. The health of mitochondria has been linked with conditions such as chronic fatigue syndrome[24].

A process known as mitochondrial biogenesis is the creation of new mitochondria. Increasing the number of mitochondria that you have (thus increasing mitochondrial density) particularly in your muscles, helps you to metabolize more fat and glucose.

Research shows that to maximize your mitochondrial density you need to include short intense forms of exercise. Incorporating a few Tabata workouts per week will help with this. One thing you can also do as part of your strength or aerobic workout is to perform a few short intense sets of cardiovascular work such as sprints (duration of 30 seconds). Research suggests that including four sets of 30 seconds of all out cycling sprints activate mitochondrial biogenesis in the skeletal muscle tissue of humans. It has also been shown that 3 sets of 5 x 4 second treadmill sprints with 20 seconds of rest in between sprints performed three times a week, has the same effect.

To enhance mitochondrial health, try adding in one or a combination of the following workouts each week:

- 4 to 6 x 30-second all out sprints on a stationary bike with 4 minutes of rest in between three times weekly, or
- 5 x 4 second treadmill sprints with 20 seconds rest in between performed three times per week.

---

24 Chronic fatigue syndrome goes beyond the scope of this book but for more on this see the work of Dr Sarah Myhill - https://www.drmyhill.co.uk/.

FLEXIBILITY AND RANGE OF MOVEMENT

Another consequence of ageing which many people seem to just accept as natural and unavoidable is a decline in range of movement and/or flexibility. Again, it doesn't have to be this way. In fact, using your days off from exercise to engage in some yoga, stretching or mobility work is a great way to schedule active recovery sessions and enhance these important areas. Most people under the age of 40 benefit from one day off from exercise per week, and those over the age of 40 from two days per week. By a day off, I don't mean sitting on the sofa bingeing on Netflix, but instead engaging in active recovery such as a longer walk, a yoga session, some stretching and mobility work, foam rolling, a sauna session or a deep tissue massage.

One of the most important times to move your body is after a night of sleep. Going for a walk, engaging in yoga or some simple sun salutations can be a great way to move your body, improve blood flow and prepare your mind and body for the day ahead. Another form of training that can be great for enhancing mobility and posture is Foundation Training created by Dr Eric Goodman. To learn more about this, I highly recommend his book 'True To Form' or downloading the 'Foundation Training' app on your phone .

This may sound like a lot to fit in at first but actually it's pretty straightforward. The first thing I would recommend is setting a time on your phone so that you remind yourself to move regularly throughout the day. Setting a timer to move every 20 to 30 minutes will help to optimise your productivity and improve your overall movement patterns. The second thing is to wake up 20 minutes earlier so that you can schedule some daily movement whether that's a walk, a yoga session or simply a few sun salutations (or if you have more time, a swim or cycle). It's amazing how powerful this routine is in setting you up with a positive outlook for the day.

There are many resources online for workouts and challenges. The main thing is to choose forms of exercise that you enjoy so that you actually do it and build consistency. Once every 2 weeks set aside 30 minutes to plan your weekly exercise sessions.

As you now know, muscle is an organ of longevity and so the first 2-3 exercise sessions you schedule into your week should be resistance training sessions. Over time, mix up the stimulus and type of exercises to avoid the SAID Principle.

MEN V WOMEN: CIRCADIAN & ULTRADIAN CYCLES

One of the key differences between men and women is that men are largely operating on the basis of their circadian rhythm i.e. the 24-hour clock whereas women have another infradian clock that works alongside the circadian clock. Women's menstrual cycle influences their physiology in many ways. Recent research shows that women's physical performance varies throughout the month. To put it simply, women have two hormone phases each month; a high hormone phase and a low hormone phase. It is during the low hormone phase that women are physiologically most similar to men in the way that they metabolize carbohydrates and recover from exertion. In the second phase of the menstrual cycle when hormones rise, it's a different story.

> As High Performance Health podcast guest, Stacy T. Sims, PHD, writes in her book ***'Roar: How To Match Your Food And Fitness To Your Female Physiology For Optimum Performance, Great Health And A Strong, Lean Body For Life'***, high oestrogen causes us to spare glycogen and increase the amount of fat we use for fuel. This makes high intensity exercise much harder to do as it uses much more glycogen (the stored carbohydrate in your body). In addition to this, higher levels of progesterone causes increases in:

- core body temperature
- sweat response
- sodium loss
- muscle breakdown.

Not only does it increase muscle breakdown but progesterone also inhibits a woman's ability to synthesise muscle since amino acids (the building blocks of protein) are not as easy to access.

Dr Stacy Sims explains that during this high-hormone phase, exercise often feels hotter than usual, particularly in the few days before menstruation as during this phase fluids shift into the cells, blood plasma volume decreases and women are more predisposed to central nervous system fatigue. In her book, Dr Sims explains that women have unique recovery needs and thus need to fuel differently to men before and during exercise.

PHYSIOLOGICAL DIFFERENCES BETWEEN MEN AND WOMEN

Muscle

Both men and women have approximately the same percentage of type I endurance (aerobic) and type II power (anaerobic) muscle fibres. The difference is that in women's bodies, the largest fibres tend to be type I endurance fibres while in men they tend to be type II power fibres. Women tend to carry more of their muscle tissue below the waist too. It may be for this reason that women seem to respond well to supersets or circuit style training with higher numbers of repetitions and shorter intervals when building muscle. Men on the other hand will often respond better to a lower rep range, with heavier weights and longer rest periods.

The most common thing I hear from women is "I don't want to get big" and "won't weight training make me look bulkier?" The answer to both of these questions and many of the other permutations is a resounding "no". In fact, strength training is absolutely fundamental to fat loss and to maintaining a lean and healthy body over your lifetime.

Fat

There are two types of fat that we store in our bodies; essential fats and storage fat. Essential fat in men is between 3 to 4% of body mass and in women it's around 12%. The key reason for this difference is that women have breasts which are largely fatty tissue, and women are also designed to reproduce. How much fat men and women carry for the most part depends on their lifestyle and nutrition, but there are also three distinct body types that play a role:

- Endomorphs - tend to be larger and carry more body fat. They are also able to build muscle more easily

- Ectomorphs - tend to be naturally slimmer and more wiry, but have a harder time building muscle
- Mesomorphs - are a blend of the other two and who tend to be lean and naturally muscular.

Lung Capacity

Women have a smaller heart and smaller lungs than men, with approximately 25 to 30% less lung capacity than men. Women also have lower diastolic pressure which is the pressure in the arteries when the heart is resting between beats. This predisposes women to have lower maximum heart rates and increased problems with dehydration in heat. Women's hearts pump out less oxygenated blood with every beat; this is estimated to be about 30% less than men. Less oxygenated blood means that women have to breathe more often than men and as a result their respiratory muscles work harder and use more energy.

In the same way that skeletal muscles need to be strong enough to perform the right contractions, the respiratory muscles need enough blood flow to facilitate the contractions to meet oxygen demand. Generally speaking women have a lower VO2 max than men. VO2 Max is the maximum amount of oxygen that your body can use to make fuel. Women's VO2 Max tends to be between 15 to 25% lower than men. If a male and female athlete are doing the same amount of work, the woman's heart rate is likely to be higher and she will need more oxygen to perform the exercise.

HORMONES

Oestrogen & Progesterone - the primary female hormones

Higher oestrogen levels mean that women tend to use more fat and less glycogen during exercise. This makes it harder for women to hit high intensities. Higher oestrogen also means that women have higher levels of body fat and lower levels of lean mass. As mentioned previously, women also tend to have smaller type II muscle fibres and the energy producing enzymes that go with those fibres. This means that they have a lower glycolytic capacity than men. What this means in practice is that when training at anaerobic threshold (in the absence of oxygen) men are more able to burn through glucose than women.

Higher oestrogen means that women find it harder to make muscle and so, during the high hormone phase of the menstrual cycle it can be harder to rebuild and repair muscles after exercise. This is compounded by the fact that higher levels of progesterone in the second phase of the menstrual cycle increase muscle breakdown. This means that getting sufficient protein post exercise is very important for women to rebuild their muscles and counter signalling by the body to store fat. Women should aim to consume between 20 to 25 g of protein within 30 minutes of finishing their exercise session.

While this is an ongoing area of research, in the second phase of the menstrual cycle it is harder for women to make and maintain muscle.

Testosterone - the primary male hormone

Men generally have higher levels of testosterone. Testosterone encourages protein synthesis and larger muscles. This also in turn leads to bigger bones. Women tend to suffer a greater loss in bone density with age. In the United States, 80% of people with osteoporosis are women. For more on bone density see the section on bone mass below.

Because of these differences between men and menstruating women, it tends to be the case that women may need to exercise slightly differently to men across the month. In fact, if women try to push themselves hard every day, and ignore many of the signs they get from fluctuating hormones, they may actually hinder their ability to get or stay lean and healthy.

Alisa Vitti, women's hormone and functional nutrition expert, bestselling author of ***'WomanCode'*** and ***'In The Flow'*** (and my guest on High Performance Health) explains that due to the rise and fall in hormones at different times of the menstrual cycle, they are more suited to certain types of training than others.

You may remember learning about the menstrual cycle in your high school biology class, but here is a quick recap. A women's cycle generally varies between 28 and 35 days in length.

The textbook 28 day day cycle look something like this:

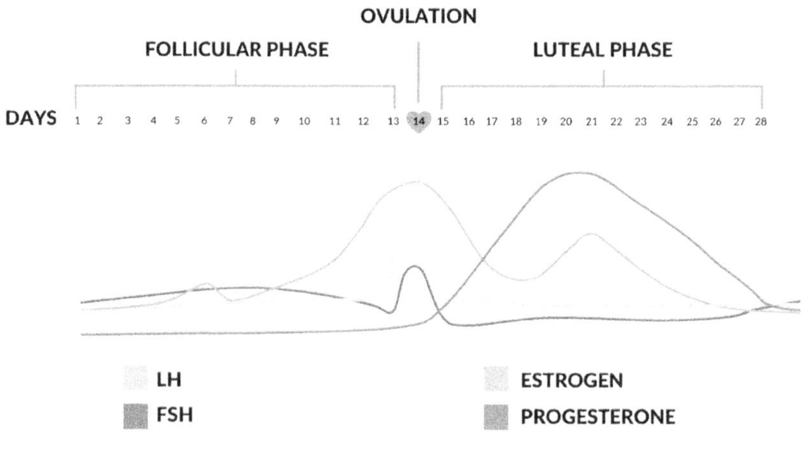

Days 1 to 14 are called the follicular phase and days 15 to 28 are the luteal phase, with ovulation occurring in the middle of the cycle. Menstruation begins on day 1 and lasts between 3 and 7 days. During menstruation, there is a rise in follicle-stimulating hormone (FSH) which helps the ovaries to mature eggs ready for release. Around day 5 or 6, the ovaries start to increase production of oestrogen and at approximately day 12 (it varies from woman to woman depending on the length of her cycle), luteinizing hormone (LH) surges causing ovulation. Oestrogen levels momentarily dip before rising again as the body prepares for a possible pregnancy. Progesterone levels rise and surpass oestrogen which prepares the lining of the uterus for implantation. Approximately 5 days before menstruation, estrogen and progesterone levels peak and some women experience symptoms of premenstrual syndrome (PMS). If pregnancy has not taken place (i.e. no egg has been fertilised) progesterone levels fall and a period takes place as the lining of the uterus is shed.

Menstrual Phase (3-7 days)

During this phase hormones are at their lowest. Energy levels vary and so women should go with what they feel in deciding whether to exercise or not. Some women experience a drop in energy and benefit from focussing on active recovery and restorative activities such as gentle yoga, pilates, breathwork and tai chi. Other women experience high energy and find that their hormones are more favourable for performance. Dr Stacy Sims says "As ironic as it may seem, your exercise physiology is most like a man's during your period and the days that follow".

The number of studies done on women and their menstrual cycles are few in number. A study of swimmers found they achieved their fastest times during menstruation and their slowest times during their premenstrual period. Paula Radcliffe broke the record for the fastest marathon in 2002 in Chicago while she had menstrual cramps. Women's achievement in endurance sports may be less affected by their period as the research shows that endurance performance indicators such as lactate threshold (the point at which your muscles burn from lactate accumulating faster than you can clear it) and VO2 Max (the maximum rate of oxygen consumption) are consistent across the menstrual cycle.

Follicular Phase (7-10 days)

The follicular phase usually lasts between 7-10 days and follows the end of your period. Estrogen, progesterone and testosterone are all lower during this phase. It is also during this stage of the menstrual cycle that women burn fat more easily and find it easier to gain muscle.

Example types of workout to do during this phase would be spin classes, running, cycling, dancing, circuit training and any other HIIT workout.

Ovulatory Phase (3-4 days)

During the ovulatory phase, estrogen and testosterone peak. This is the time to crush that workout or possibly to achieve a personal best! The types of workouts suited to ovulation are intense workouts such as interval sprint training, HIIT or kickboxing.

Luteal Phase (10-14 days)

In this phase women have a faster metabolism and generally burn more calories than the beginning of the month. Higher levels of oestrogen reduce their ability to burn carbohydrates while increasing fat burning and fatty acid availability. When doing high intensity training during this stage it will likely be necessary to eat more carbohydrates. This may also explain why many women crave more carbs during the high hormone phase of their cycle and during PMS. Studies show that women experience a 5-10% increase in metabolic rate in the days leading up to their period.

In the first 5 days of the luteal phase, estrogen and testosterone are still relatively high, but as this phase progresses these levels drop while progesterone rises. A 2003 study in Sports Medicine found that women reach exhaustion faster in the mid-luteal phase compared to the first half of the cycle. They are also more likely to be injured during this phase and menstruation.

Rising levels of progesterone are catabolic and so it is harder to gain muscle. Hard workouts can aggravate this and may thwart efforts to gain muscle and lose fat.

Strength training can be a good option in the first five days of this phase, but lower intensity training is advised as energy levels will likely be diminishing. For the last 5-10 days of this phase, it may be better to engage in more gentle activities such as yoga, pilates or barre.

Exercise is likely to feel harder in the high hormone phase. Ignoring this and pushing through raises cortisol and can make the body more likely to gain fat and catabolize muscle. When estrogen and progesterone levels are high it can make it harder for women to cool in hotter temperatures or longer aerobic sessions compared to men. This is particularly the case as women generally begin to sweat later into a workout. Higher progesterone also raises core body temperature and lowers blood volume which means that it's harder to sweat and cool the body during this stage. Progesterone also increases the loss of sodium which increases your risk of heat stress in endurance events in hotter climates.

During this high hormone phase, apart from exercise feeling harder it is also harder to build muscle. Higher levels of estrogen and progesterone have a big impact on muscle-cell turnover and protein synthesis. High estrogen lowers the ability to grow muscle while high progesterone increases muscle breakdown. This means that during hard workouts higher levels of muscle mass break down. As such,it's not just harder to make muscle during the high hormone phase but also harder to maintain muscle when estrogen and progesterone are high.

Some of this can be offset by making sure that there is enough protein in the diet, particularly after exercise. Whey protein or an essential amino acid blend are good sources to refuel with especially as they contain leucine which is the muscle building amino acid. One third of muscle tissue is made of branched chain amino acids (leucine, isoleucine and valine). More on this in Chapter 4.

Beat the Bloat

Do you struggle to get into your skinny jeans right before your period? Perhaps you feel as though you may have gained a few pounds?

There are reasons for this. High estrogen and progesterone affect the hormones that regulate fluid levels in your body.

Progesterone competes for the same receptor site with aldosterone which regulates sodium. With the competition of progesterone, less aldosterone is released which leads to a reduction in blood volume. Higher estrogen levels lead to an increase in the hormone vasopressin which is responsible for retaining water and constricting blood vessels. This leads to the body retaining water and constricting blood vessels to some degree. This results in the bloated and sluggish feeling.

Just as you are experiencing PMS symptoms and feeling lower in energy and mood, you may be experiencing carb cravings while simultaneously feeling as though you've gained weight all of a sudden. The temptation is to push harder, increase your intermittent fasting window, add in more HIIT, drop carb intake and generally overstress your body in your quest to stay lean and capitalise on the results you've achieved to this point in the month.

Note to women, this is where it is time to rethink...

Women may be better off going with the flow of they feel, focussing on gentler activities like yoga, tai chi, a swim or a hike. This is not necessarily the time to be trying to gain muscle or hit a PB. Higher estrogen levels mean it is harder to build muscle. On top of this, higher progesterone levels mean women catabolise (break down) muscle more easily. Women's metabolic rate is higher so they will be burning more energy (approximately 150-200 extra calories per day). Keep active with all day movement and give yourself a well earned break. This is the ideal time for women to work on often neglected areas such as flexibility, foam rolling, mobility and postural work. Or treat yourself to a full body massage.

Your body and mind will thank you!

HOW HEALTHY IS YOUR BONE BANK?

Many people assume that a loss in bone density is something that only women need to worry about. It's true that bone density loss is an issue for many post-menopausal women, who comprise 80% of people in the United States with osteoporosis. But to think that it's only women that need to look after their bones would be a mistake.

Most people think of bones as a static structure. In reality bones are constantly being remodelled - your body absorbs old bone and creates new bone in its place. As a result of higher testosterone levels, men have both bigger muscles and bigger bones which means their bone mass is greater. Both men and women hit their peak bone mass between the ages of 30 and 35. After the age of 35, bone breakdown starts to outpace bone rebuilding. The rate of bone loss in pre-menopausal women is between 0.5-1% percent each year. Estrogen levels help with bone remodelling but after menopause, bone loss can accelerate to a loss rate of 2-3% per year. Some of this bone loss is genetic and you can discover with a DNA test if you are likely to be susceptible.

There are also some important things that both men and women should do to preserve bone density.

The first and most important thing you can do is, you guessed it, move more! Every time you move, your muscles pull on your bones to create the movement. The cells within your bones sense the stress and respond by making your bones stronger and more dense. The types of exercises you should be doing to strengthen your bones are:

- Weight bearing activities - a minimum of 2-3 times per week. These should include strength training with additional resistance, or using your body weight which requires you to work against the force of gravity

- Moderate impact activities - such as walking, running, ball sports or dancing. While swimming and cycling are great for your heart, they don't do so much for your bones.

If you are someone that has already been diagnosed with osteopenia or osteoporosis then it is probably best to avoid high impact activities such as plyometrics or anything that involves lots of twisting and bending which can place too much pressure on your spinal vertebrae.

Studies of postmenopausal women with low bone density saw around 1% gains in the density of their spine and hip bones with regular strength training. Tai chi is also a great form of exercise, especially for people with thinning bones as it strengthens the entire lower body and improves balance which makes you less likely to fall.

Postural exercises are particularly important, especially exercises for the upper back as these help to strengthen the muscles in your thoracic spine between your shoulder blades. This in turn helps to reduce rounding of the shoulders which places undue stress on the spinal column. Over time this kind of stress can lead to compression fractures. This is especially important for women who have less muscle mass and consequently thinner bones in their upper body.

Men and women over the age of 65 should have their bone density measured. Some individuals should have this checked earlier particularly those who:

- have a family history of osteoporosis
- have DNA test results indicating they are at risk
- have used medication such as glucocorticosteroids that are known to impair bone health
- have reason to suspect they may suffer from bone density issues.

RETHINK > > >

TRADITIONAL THINKING:

- We can expect to slowly lose strength as we age with very little we can do about it.
- As we age, our metabolism slows down and gradually weight gain is inevitable.
- The same exercise guidelines apply to men and menstruating women.

RETHINK:

- We can maintain healthy body composition and bone density throughout our lives by training and moving intelligently.
- Humans were not born to sit, but rather to move regularly.
- We need to move at least every hour and combine different forms of movement and exercise over the course of each and every week to ensure that we maintain muscle mass, flexibility, mobility, cardiovascular health and metabolic flexibility.
- We should walk a lot, run sometimes and lift heavy things a few times each week.

Your brain and body will thank you for it.

For more resources on how to optimise physical fitness, in particular how to optimise your training according to your genetics (which has been scientifically validated to give 3 times the results, but is beyond the scope of this book) go to www.rethinkhealth.club.

Chapter 4
MASTER YOUR NUTRITION

"Let food be thy medicine and medicine be thy food"
Hypocrates

The poet Lucretius wrote "one man's meat is another man's poison". He meant this in the broader sense, not just in relation to food, but it certainly holds true for food as well.

Take nuts for example. For some people these are a great source of healthy fats, protein, vitamins and antioxidants like vitamin E. For others they can trigger anaphylactic shock and prove to be fatal. The average person may tolerate a little gluten in their diet. For those individuals who are celiac, gluten damages their small intestine to such a degree that it can cause serious long term health implications.

We've all seen that person who can eat whatever they want and seemingly never gain weight or experience any digestive problems. Legend has it that Usain Bolt consumed 1000 chicken nuggets during the Beijing Olympics. The newspapers reported that he powered up with around five boxes of chicken nuggets each day, with french fries and apple pies for dessert. We're not all Usain Bolt!

You might be wondering what type of diet you should be following, and most likely have friends that thrive on one diet or another.

Social media has popularised a number of different diets recently, ranging from the Keto diet to the Carnivore diet to raw vegan. Millions of people across the world are battling with the bulge.

According to research in the New England Journal of Medicine, 42% of the US population are estimated to be obese with that figure expected to rise to 48.9% in 2030. The researchers predict that by 2030, no state will have an obesity rate below 35% and in some states the rate of obesity will hit 60%[25].

Obesity is on the increase despite us having more access to nutritional advice, documentaries and healthy eating programmes on mainstream media than ever before. The weight loss industry is booming, continuing to grow year on year.

In the United States alone, in 2019 the diet and weight loss market was worth a staggering $72 billion with a forecast growth of 2.6% annually through to 2023[26].

A large proportion of the population spend much of their life going from one diet plan to the next in the eternal search for the perfect regime. They often hear from friends and family who experienced amazing results with a particular diet and who therefore proclaim that it's the "best one"! Research shows that any diet, whether low fat, low carb, keto, DASH (Dietary Approaches to Stop Hypertension) or Meditereanean lead to moderate weight loss in the short term, but issues remain with keeping weight down in the longer term. Diets can be hard to sustain. It isn't always easy for example, to eat out on the keto diet.

In a meta-analysis[27] of 121 randomized controlled trials totalling 21,942 overweight and obese participants, researchers compared the effects of 14 popular diets on both weight loss and cardiovascular disease risk.The results showed that at 6 months, all diets had led to modest weight loss and substantial reductions in cardiovascular disease risk. However, these benefits were largely diminished at 12 months, apart from the Mediterranean diet's continued benefit to cardiovascular health. These findings suggest that any diet may be used to promote weight loss, but issues with keeping the weight down in the longer term need to be addressed.

---

25 https://www.nejm.org/doi/full/10.1056/NEJMsa1909301
26 https://blog.marketresearch.com/u.s.-weight-loss-industry-grows-to-72-billion
27 https://pubmed.ncbi.nlm.nih.gov/32238384/

Is there such a thing as a perfect diet?

As you learnt in the last chapter, It's important to have a lean and strong body, with muscle being an organ of longevity. Many people who don't fall within the overweight or obese category are still "under-muscled". Muscle mass helps to give you metabolic flexibility and better insulin sensitivity. It burns more calories than fat and so gives you more latitude if you go of course. The right body composition helps to protect you against many modern-day chronic diseases like heart disease, diabetes and cancer.

For many people, in simple terms it's about looking good, feeling good and living younger for longer.

What is the perfect diet for you? Can you truly have it all or must there be compromises and sacrifices?

The truth is, there is no perfect diet. There is no one size fits all.

But, there is a perfect diet for you.

That diet is the one that fits with your unique biology and environment.

Our bodies process the foods that we eat in different ways depending on our underlying genetics, our microbiome, our hormone levels, our lifestyle, our energy demands and our current health status. Food is a signalling molecule and it tells our body what to do. Food is information. It is not as simple as calories in versus calories out. If it were, we would most likely not be experiencing the current obesity epidemic.

Does this statement conflict with the first law of thermodynamics? In a way, yes.

The first law of thermodynamics states that the energy of an isolated system is constant. This means that in a laboratory or an isolated system, 1,000 calories of kale would release the same amount of energy as 1,000 calories of soda. However, we are not an isolated system living in a constant environment. As such, the law of thermodynamics cannot be unilaterally applied to living, breathing systems. Food is information and when you eat, your body decides what to do with that information. As New York Times bestselling author Mark Hyman MD states:

"... law of thermodynamics doesn't apply in living, breathing, digesting systems. When you eat food, the "isolated system" part of the equation goes out the window. The food interacts with your biology, a complex adaptive system that instantly transforms every bite."

Many people on the popularised ketogenic diet have reversed blood sugar problems, lost significant amounts of body fat, sharpened their focus and mental acuity and feel fantastic as a result of the diet! For others, a strict ketogenic diet could wreak havoc on their bodies with high cholesterol and atherosclerosis as a result of following it.

So how can you find the perfect diet for you?

We have evolved over tens of thousands of years depending on our ancestors and where they lived and what they ate. The perfect diet for you depends on a variety of factors which include your:

- genetics
- ancestry
- activity levels and energy demands
- stage of life
- gut health
- inflammation levels
- blood sugar regulation
- gut and the microbes in it
- intolerances and allergies
- overall health status.

Your DNA

You are uniquely you because of your genetics. Following completion of the Human Genome Project in 2004, scientists concluded that we each have around 25000 genes.

To understand this, we need a short science lesson. I promise to keep this simple.

DNA stands for **deoxyribonucleic acid**.

DNA is a chemical made up of two long molecules, arranged in a spiral called the **double-helix** structure.

A DNA molecule consists of two strands that wind around each other like a twisted ladder. Each strand has a backbone, made up of alternating groups of sugar (deoxyribose) and phosphate.

Each sugar is attached to one of four bases:

- adenine (A),
- cytosine (C),
- guanine (G)
- thymine (T)

The two strands are held together by bonds between the bases. Adenine (A) forms a base pair with Thymine (T) and Cytosine (C) forms a base pair with Guanine (G).

The nucleus in every cell in your body contains DNA, which carries genetic information about you. It has all the instructions that a living organism needs to function, grow and reproduce.

GENES

Genes are short sections of DNA. Genes carry information about particular characteristics such as eye colour or hair colour. A umber of genes together make up a chromosome.

CHROMOSOMES

In a cell nucleus, DNA is organised into coiled strands called chromosomes. Humans have 46 chromosomes in each cell, 23 of which are inherited from each parent. This explains why you might have your mother's eyes with your father's hair colour.

By looking at your genetics you can determine (for example) what your tolerance is towards carbohydrates and fats. This is important because if you have certain genetic markers, depending on your activity levels and metabolism, a strict ketogenic diet (containing a high volume of saturated fats like butter, ghee and coconut oil) could lead to elevated levels of LDL cholesterol as high as 400mg/dl, along with high levels of inflammation and raised triglyceride levels.

Individuals sometimes, but not always, get symptoms alongside this which include general tiredness or fatigue, joint pain, lowered physical performance and gastrointestinal distress.

WHAT DO YOU NEED TO BE AWARE OF BEFORE EMBARKING ON ANY SPECIFIC DIET?

Firstly you need to check your own genetics which can be as simple as a 60 second salivary test that you can do in the comfort of your own home. There are a number of companies that offer DNA testing and they range from testing arrays to whole exome sequencing. When looking at which DNA test to buy you will want to ensure that the company has strict data protection and privacy policies in place.

The data also needs to be usable by you. Companies such as 23andme give you raw data, and you can pay extra to process this through an external algorithm such as that provided by Stratagene or FoundMyFitness by Dr Rhonda Patrick which helps to understand the data and make it more usable.

Other companies provide you with a customised report automatically and give you actionable steps together with consultations on how to utilise your genetics for enhanced health and performance.

Nutrigenomics is a rapidly evolving area of science but at the time of writing, what are the key areas that you need to be paying attention to?

In the pages that follow I will outline some of the main aspects of your nutrition that you should look to personalise according to your genetics together with general principles that will help you to structure your diet for optimal body composition and longevity

THE MACRONUTRIENTS THAT MAKE UP YOUR DIET

There are 3 sources of macronutrients that make up your diet:

- Protein
- Fats
- Carbohydrates

Protein

Protein, found in larger quantities in meat, poultry, fish, dairy products, eggs, beans and pulses, is broken down by the body into amino acids. Amino acids play a role in almost every system in our body including in the creation and growth of muscles, connective tissue and skin.

Your body needs 20 different amino acids to grow and function properly. Of these amino acids, nine are classified as essential.

Essential amino acids can't be made by your body and must be obtained through your diet. The essential amino acids are histidine, isoleucine, leucine, lysine, methionine, phenylalanine, threonine, tryptophan and valine.

Protein is essential for virtually every cellular function in your body, including structure, metabolism, regulation of tissues and organs (including muscle) and synthesising thyroid hormones. It is used to make enzymes, hormones and neurotransmitters.

As you learnt in Chapter 3, muscle is very important for metabolic health and longevity. It is the foundation of your metabolism - the stronger and healthier your muscles, the better you are able to burn carbohydrates and fats. Having sufficient muscle tissue also helps you to look 'fit and toned'.

Dr Gabrielle Lyon has done a huge amount of research around protein and the importance of it to metabolism. She advises designing your meals around high quality protein. This helps to ensure that you stimulate sufficient muscle protein synthesis, especially when combined with resistance training. In eating protein, you also benefit from the thermic effect, which means that you use more energy to digest protein. It's the combination of resistance exercise with sufficient protein that gives you the muscle definition and that lean, toned look. Dieting - crash dieting and yo-yo dieting leads to weight loss, but you don't just lose fat on most of these diets, you also lose muscle. The more muscle you lose, the harder it is to get it back and get your metabolism on track. You want to regularly stimulate muscle protein synthesis.

Muscle protects you in so many ways. It helps you regulate blood sugar and manage both adipose tissue (body fat) and blood lipid levels. Muscles provide a reservoir of amino acids for your body to draw upon in times of need. Amino acids are used to synthesize new cells, proteins, antibodies and peptides for the immune response. In periods of stress, your body can draw upon your amino acid reserves to protect other vital organs such as the liver, kidney and brain.

How much protein do you need?

The current recommended daily allowance (RDA) for protein is set at 0.8grams per kg of body mass (0.36grams per pound). For a 175lb (approx. 80kg) male or 135lbs woman (approx 61kg), this would be 64g protein and 49g protein respectively. This is very low. The RDA is simply there to give you the minimum to stay alive. It does not account for individuals who want to enhance their longevity and protect against muscle loss. The RDA is not enough to build muscle and enhance proper tissue repair.

If you exercise regularly, are looking to lose weight healthily and/or protect your muscles for longevity, you need between 1.4g-2.5g per kg of bodyweight. For most people in this category, a good starting point is 1g per 1lb of bodyweight (2.2.g per kg). If you are looking to lose weight, you should adjust this figure to 1g per 1lb of your target weight.

1g x Bodyweight in lbs = Protein Daily Amount in Grams

There are three types of amino acids that warrant particular highlighting if you are looking to maintain optimal body composition. These are leucine, lysine and methionine.

Leucine

Leucine is key in driving muscle protein synthesis. It has also been shown to increase our ability to burn fatty acids[28] and is a modulator of insulin signaling. Our intake of leucine should increase as we age.

Lysine

Lysine is responsible for the proteins in your connective tissues and plays a part in collagen formation which is needed not just for your skin (so you look younger!) but also for your tendons and ligaments. Tendons are the connective tissue that connect muscle to bone and ligaments connect bones together at your joints. Lysine is also a precursor for carnitine, which transports fatty acids to the mitochondria, where they can be oxidised for the release of energy (used for fuel).

Methionine

Like lysine, methionine is important for the synthesis of carnitine and also another amino acid, cysteine. Cysteine is a precursor to glutathione which is the body's master antioxidant. Methionine is important for muscle protein synthesis and also plays a role in detoxification of heavy metals and cellular protection.

Animal sources contain the highest amounts of these three amino acids with the highest amounts of all three being present in chicken, beef and yellowfin tuna. If you follow a vegan diet you may want

28 https://pubmed.ncbi.nlm.nih.gov/26255285/

to think about supplementing with an essential amino acid blend.

Branch chain amino acids (BCAAs) namely leucine, isoleucine and valine have also been shown to support muscle growth and boost exercise performance. However, I prefer to take essential amino acids rather than BCAAs for a few reasons:

- A good essential amino acid blend contains all of the BCAAs in the correct ratios
- High doses of BCAAs on their own can deplete levels of B vitamins. The enzymes required to break down and use BCAAs require B vitamins as cofactors and so taking high doses can eventually disrupt many of the other processes that rely on B vitamins. If you want healthy hair, skin and nails, good levels of energy from proper breakdown of food, optimised hormonal and neurotransmitter function and proper DNA repair and methylation then it's probably safer to stick to essential amino acids.
- BCAAs may affect glucose metabolism and contribute to insulin resistance when taken in high amounts.
- Lower mood and lethargy - when levels of BCAAs are high, there is less uptake of tryptophan by the brain as both of these are transported by the same carrier system. Lower levels of tryptophan can lead to lower production of serotonin (a calming and relaxing neurotransmitter that boosts mood and also helps you produce enough melatonin to sleep well).

Fats

There are three types of fats: saturated, monounsaturated and polyunsaturated fats.

Saturated Fats

Saturated fats are composed of single bonded carbon atoms which are saturated with hydrogen. Saturated fats are solid at room temperature and are found in red meat, whole fat dairy foods, cheese and coconut oil.

Monounsaturated fats (MUFAs):

Monounsaturated fats have one double bond in the fatty acid chain with all of the remainder single bonded carbon atoms.

Examples of monounsaturated fats are olive oil, peanut oil, canola oil, avocados, and most nuts as well as high-oleic safflower and sunflower oils.

Polyunsaturated fats (PUFAs):

Polyunsaturated fats have at least two double carbon bonds. They are essential fats. This means that they are required for normal body functions but your body is not able to make them. You need to obtain polyunsaturated fats from food. Polyunsaturated fats are used to build cell membranes and the covering of nerves. They are also required for blood clotting, muscle movement, and reduction of inflammation.

There are two main types of polyunsaturated fats: omega-3 and omega-6. Sources of omega-6 are oils of vegetables such as sunflower, soybean, walnut, corn and safflower. Many people consume too many omega-6 oils as they are contained within a lot of processed foods such as cookies, pastries, crisps and french fries. The ideal ratio of omega-3 to omega-6 fats is somewhere between 1:3 and 1:4 although the Standard American Diet is somewhere closer to 1:15. This has been correlated with a pro-inflammatory profile.

Polyunsaturated fats are also easily oxidised and so care should be taken to ensure that you are consuming the highest quality fats that have not been exposed to high temperatures which can easily turn them rancid.

The minimum amount of essential fats needed is around 3 grams per day. To get this amount of essential fats we need to consume a minimum of 25-30% of our total calories from fats. To work out the amount of fats that you need, you can use this simple calculation:

0.4g x bodyweight in lbs = daily essential fats requirement in g.

Healthy sources of omega-3 fatty acids include fatty fish such as salmon, mackerel,sardines, herrings, flaxseeds and walnuts.

Omega-3 fatty acids may help to prevent heart disease and strokes. Omega-3s have been shown to reduce blood pressure, raise HDL and lower triglycerides. Evidence also suggests omega-3 fats may help to reduce the need for corticosteroid medications in people with rheumatoid arthritis.[29]

Once you have calculated your macronutrient requirements for protein and fats, then you can look at either adding in additional fats (if, for example, you are following the ketogenic diet) and/or carbohydrates according to your total caloric needs. Total caloric needs will be based on your resting metabolic rate (the number of calories needed to perform your body's most basic (basal) functions like breathing, circulation and cell production) plus your additional requirements to account for extra calories burned through daily activities and exercise.

Basal metabolic rate can be measured in a laboratory setting or estimated using the Harris Benedict Equation:

Men:

BMR = 88.362 + (13.397 x weight in kg) + (4.799 x height in cm) - (5.677 x age in years)

Women:

BMR = 447.593 + (9.247 x weight in kg) + (3.098 x height in cm) - (4.330 x age in years)

29 https://www.health.harvard.edu/staying-healthy/the-truth-about-fats-bad-and-good

Deduct the total amount of calories for protein and essential fats to give you the remaining calories. You will then need to add additional calories on top according to your lifestyle, body composition goals and physical activity levels. As we all process carbohydrates and fats differently depending on a variety of factors including our gut microbiome, our genetics, our hormone levels and our physical activity and lifestyle demands, it is worth working with a health professional to do this.

Carbohydrates

Carbohydrates are the sugars, starches and fibers found in fruits, grains, vegetables and milk products. There is no such thing as an 'essential carbohydrate' although most health professionals agree that we do need fibre and highly active individuals will most likely need a greater number of total calories in their diet.

All carbohydrates are broken down into simple sugars. How quickly they are broken down depends on the type of carbohydrate - whether it is a simple carbohydrate or a complex carbohydrate. Complex carbohydrates such as quinoa, brown rice, barley and oats are broken down more slowly than simple carbohydrates such as white bread, rice and pasta.

All vegetables and fruit contain carbohydrates and the fibre contained within them can help to slow down the release, resulting in less blood sugar spikes. Tropical fruits such as grapes, mangoes and cherries are higher in sugar than raspberries, strawberries and avocados. How many carbohydrates you should include in your diet comes down to a few factors which include:

- your genetics and how quickly you process carbohydrates
- your energy demands in terms of lifestyle and fitness demands

- your metabolism
- your stress levels
- your size
- your age

Like protein, carbohydrates contain around 4 calories per gram. After you have worked out the amount of protein and fats you need to include in your diet, the remaining calories should comprise healthy forms of carbohydrates in the form of vegetables, fruits, beans and lentils and, if you can digest them, whole grains. Many forms of grains need to be soaked, sprouted or fermented to be properly digestible. For a good resource on how to do this, read 'Nourishing Traditions' by Sally Fallon.

AVOID PROCESSED FOODS

A very important part of any nutritional programme is that you should avoid, or at the very least drastically limit processed foods in your diet. Processed foods typify the Standard American Diet which is full of refined grains, stripped of their essential nutrients and often combined with additional sugar, fat and salt. The effect of this? The food becomes hyperpalatable - irresistible to eat and it is difficult to tell when you are full! They are almost impossible to eat in moderation. If you look to Mother Nature, you'll find it difficult to identify many whole foods that combine large amounts of sugar or starch with fat. We tend to find sugary foods in the form of fruits and fattier foods in the form of nuts, seeds, dairy products, meat and fish. Milk and coconuts are the few examples of foods that have sugar and fat combined.

Processed foods also often contain vegetable oils which can be rancid and highly oxidised. As you will read later in this chapter, processed vegetable oils are high in omega-6 fatty acids which can throw off your ratio of omega-6 to omega-3 fats and heighten inflammation.

On top of this, the high amounts of refined sugars in many processed foods lead to poor blood sugar control which stokes the inflammatory fire further and over time, can lead to insulin resistance.

Many of the chronic diseases that we are seeing today including heart disease, cancer and diabetes have been associated with high levels of inflammation and poor blood sugar control.

Processed foods are also very calorie dense and this, combined with their hyperpalatable nature and inflammatory profile provides the perfect storm for increased weight gain.

In research by the National institutes of Health[30] scientists saw firsthand the effect of eating a highly processed diet. This study involved a group of people who over time, were given processed foods in the form of crisps (potato chips), fruit juice and bagels with cream cheese or perishable fresh whole foods. When the individuals were eating whole unprocessed foods, they ate until they were full and effortlessly achieved weight loss. When they ate the processed foods, they were less satiated and ate more calories. The average daily energy surplus was 508 calories per day, mostly from carbohydrates and fats. 508 calories per day quickly adds up to approximately 1lb of stored fat each week!

It's no wonder that the number of people that are overweight and obese is rising so rapidly. A study published in the December 19, 2019, issue of the New England Journal of Medicine predicts that by 2030 in 29 States across the USA more than half of the population will be obese and all states will have obesity rates higher than 35%. The researchers estimated that currently, 40% of American adults are obese with 18% being severly obese. [31]In the United Kingdom, the situation is not that much different. As of 2019, 28.7% of adults in England were obese with a further 35.6% overweight. When you couple this with the fact that according to Cancer Research UK, being overweight or obese is the second biggest cause of cancer, we are clearly becoming a very sick population.

Obesity and being overweight is a complex problem with multi factoral roots that can arise from a combination of social, economic and emotional drivers. To lose weight we need to get healthier in the first place and it's the combination of factors in this book from optimising your sleep, your nutrition, your movement, your stress and your lifestyle that will help you get you there.

If there is one thing that you take away from this chapter on nutrition, let it be this- make the mainstay of your diet whole,

30 https://www.cell.com/cell-metabolism/pdf/S1550-4131(19)30248-7.pdf
31 https://www.hsph.harvard.edu/news/press-releases/half-of-us-to-have-obesity-by-2030/

unprocessed foods. Let me say that again - make the mainstay of your diet whole, unprocessed foods. Getting the proportion of protein, fats, fibre and carbohydrates right for you is covered in the sections that follow, but if you remove processed foods and make whole unprocessed foods the mainstay of your diet, you will go a long way towards optimising the health of your body and mind.

My aim with this chapter is not to give you a diet plan, but rather to teach you how different foods affect different people. I want to help you to make the right choices for your body and mind so that you can eat in a way that minimises your risk of chronic diseases, gives you a strong body and a clear and focussed mind.

Crowd out the 'bad food'

The best way to do this is crowd out the bad foods with foods that are nourishing for your body and mind. There are so many different nutritional plans out there from the carnivore diet, the keto diet, pescetarian diets, blood type diets, vegetarian, vegan and more. Each person is different and will suit a different ratio of macronutrients depending on their metabolism, genetics, spiritual practices, food preferences, lifestyle demands, location and many other factors. However, ensuring that you are getting enough protein and essential fats together with fibre is key.

I mentioned earlier how to calculate your total caloric needs and ratios. Many people eat more than enough carbohydrates but are not getting enough fibre. Fibre is important for healthy bowel movements and soluble fibre (found in apples, citrus fruits and oats) may also help to decrease your total blood cholesterol. A healthy amount of fibre is to consume 14g for every 1000 calories you eat. High fibre, low sugar foods include vegetables, beans, lentils and berries.

The Blue Zones - areas of the world with the highest number of centenarians who are mostly free of chronic disease, teach us that a diverse range of diets can keep us healthy, disease-free and help us to live a long time. In Okinawa, the population's diet is centered around fish, rice and tubers. This is naturally lower in fat, not because they are eating processed low fat foods but because their local whole foods are naturally low in fat. In contrast, the Masai incorporate meat, milk and blood from their cattle.

To optimise your diet, you need to focus on including:

- fibrous vegetables such as leafy greens and cruciferous vegetables (broccoli, bok choy, cauliflower),
- low sugar fruits (such as berries, avocado, apples and citrus fruits)
- grass-fed, free range sources of protein such as grass fed beef and lamb, free range chicken, pasture raised pork and wild, oily fish)
- healthy fats such as cold pressed extra virgin olive oil, grass fed butter, nuts and seeds

KEEP CARBS LOW FOR HIGH FOCUS AND CONCENTRATION

One of the key things that many people find is that by keeping their intake of carbohydrates low, they can stabilise their blood sugar levels effectively and improve focus and concentration. This also helps with staying naturally lean and keeping body fat within a healthy range provided that you are eating sufficient levels of protein.

When you eat, cortisol levels naturally rise. A high carbohydrate intake also leads to blood sugar levels rising and falling more rapidly leaving you feeling hungrier and sometimes struggling with food cravings. This can cause larger spikes in cortisol and also send you on a blood sugar roller coaster which makes concentration harder. See the diagram below for a visual representation of how this works.

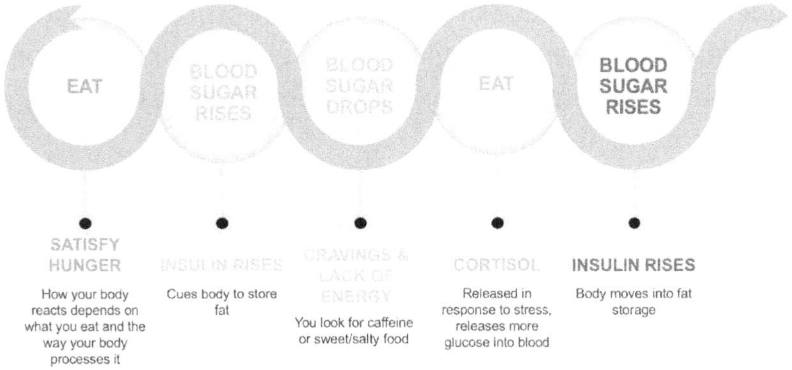

Unless you are moving a lot and have a very active job (like my tennis coach, for example who covers anywhere between 30,000 and 40,000 steps per day on his tracker) you probably don't need all of those carbohydrates that you're eating.

Whenever levels of sugar in the blood are elevated, the pancreas releases a hormone called insulin. Insulin helps to move blood sugar into the cells of the liver and muscles and helps to bring your blood sugar back down to its normal level. The liver and muscles can only hold a limited amount of long-term glucose (known as glycogen) following which the excess sugar is converted into triglycerides and can be stored as body fat (adipose tissue). When insulin levels are consistently high over a long period of time cells can become tolerant to insulin. When this happens, insulin is not able to efficiently clear sugar from the blood which can cause blood sugar levels to be elevated for extended periods. This contributes to inflammation which can damage blood vessels across your body including those that supply the brain and other organs.

Insulin is also a type of growth hormone and helps to create an environment that favours fat storage. If you find that you are gaining weight around your abdominal area (known as visceral fat) you are most likely not managing your blood sugar terribly well.

When insulin is high, it also blocks your ability to burn fat. In modern times, because of the number of processed foods in our diet, many people are struggling with higher insulin levels for much of the time and consequently carry more body fat than they would like and than is healthy.

In addition, it may surprise you to learn that many of our organs actually like to burn fat for fuel. Your heart muscle is designed to obtain 40 to 70% of its energy from fat. Your supercomputer, the brain (which utilises glucose very effectively) can also be powered by fat. Fatty acids are converted by the liver into compounds known as ketone bodies (or ketones). When ketones are present and you have entered a natural state known as ketosis, they can help to increase the production of gamma-aminobutyric acid (GABA), a neurotransmitter that exerts a calming effect on the brain. This is one of the main reasons that a ketogenic diet is so effective in helping to treat epilepsy.

Ketones also help to increase the expression of brain-derived neurotrophic factor (BDNF). BDNF is an amazing protein that helps to promote the growth of new cells in the hippocampus (the brain's memory centre). In this way, by raising levels of BDNF, ketones may help to support neuroplasticity, the brain's ability to reorganize itself by forming new neural connections throughout life. Increasing production of BDNF is a powerful anti-aging hack!

It's for this reason that many individuals prefer to consume a moderated cyclical ketogenic style diet with added greens for fibre. This involves eating mostly protein and healthy fats with some fibrous vegetables during the day and saving a small dose of carbohydrates for the evening meal. As you learnt in the chapter on sleep, this can help to facilitate a good night's sleep. This style of eating helps to boost mental clarity and function so that you can get your best work done, while helping to reduce inflammation and simultaneously assist in achieving your body composition goals. Cycling in and out of mild ketosis in this way can also help to preserve proper thyroid function.

Many people also find that not eating at all for most of the day helps with concentration and body composition goals. Diet plans such as the 16:8 or 20:4 regimes involve fasting for 16-20 hours and compressing the eating window to 4-8 hours. Depending on your lifestyle demands, this isn't necessarily right for everyone and personally I would find it difficult to eat enough protein and fat within a four window without feeling uncomfortable. The idea with these types of intermittent fasts is not to reduce the total amount of food (although estimates suggest total calorie intake does naturally reduce), but simply to compress the eating window.

Fasting for extended periods may not be the best option for menstruating women as it can interfere with hormonal balance. For busy women in their menstruating years who exercise frequently and are busy working and taking care of children and a home, for example, it can add too much stress if regularly fasting for more than 12-14 hours a day.

It's true that fasting or ketogenesis (see below) can help with a process known as autophagy during which old and worn out cells get recycled. Being in a fed state is also important as this too is associated with repair protection and rebuilding. It is for this reason that for men, in particular, who do not have the same hormonal concerns as menstruating women, I encourage a minimum 12 to 14 hour overnight fast with a mildly ketogenic state during the day and a refeed with carbohydrates in the evening.

WHAT IS A KETOGENIC DIET?

The ketogenic diet is an extremely high-fat, low-carb diet. It is championed by many who swear by it as the ideal way to lose weight and enhance cognition. It's also a diet commonly used by endurance athletes such as triathletes and cyclists. Many people take exogenous ketones to help them enter ketosis more quickly and this can be a great strategy especially if you have a particularly cognitively demanding day ahead.

Is the keto diet right for everyone? As with all things nutritional, we return to the fact that it is highly individual. For some people, following a strict ketogenic diet can lead to worryingly high levels of LDL cholesterol, together with high levels of triglycerides (which can be a risk factor for heart disease) and also higher levels of inflammation. Sometimes (but not always) these people will experience anxiety, fatigue, joint pain and lowered levels of physical performance as well.

WHAT IS THE CORRECT PROPORTION OF FATS AND SATURATED FATS IN YOUR DIET?

Every day we seem to read something different about fats. From statements like "saturated fats are harmful" to the polar opposite of putting butter in your morning cup of Joe and following a ketogenic diet, it seems confusing at best, as to how many saturated fats you should eat. You've probably also heard that "high cholesterol is bad for you" and more and more people are being prescribed statins. According to John Hopkins Medical School, more than 200 million people across the world take statins.

What is Cholesterol?

Cholesterol is a waxy, fat-like substance that is produced in the body and is also obtained from consuming foods that come from animals (particularly egg yolks, meat, poultry, fish, and dairy products).

Cholesterol is actually needed by the body to build cell membranes, make certain hormones, and produce compounds that help digest fat.

Health issues can arise when individuals have excess cholesterol circulating that they are not able to get rid of and so it builds up in the blood. Too much cholesterol increases a person's risk of developing heart disease. This happens more often in people with familial hypercholesterolemia.

Familial Hypercholesterolemia

This is an inherited genetic condition that is characterized by very high levels of cholesterol in the blood. It is thought to affect up to ten percent of the world's population.

Individuals with familial hypercholesterolemia have an elevated risk of developing coronary artery disease at a young age.

The coronary arteries supply blood to the heart. Excess cholesterol can end up deposited on the inner walls of the blood vessels in the arteries and starts to form clumps (plaques) that narrow the arteries and also harden the artery walls. As these plaques build up and get bigger, they can start to clog the arteries and result in restricted blood flow to the heart. This places the individual at a higher risk of heart attack and may also cause an associated type of chest pain called angina.

In individuals with familial hypercholesterolemia (FH) the excess cholesterol can also build up in tissues other than the heart and blood vessels. It can build up in the tissues that attach muscles to bones (tendons), with fatty deposits around the elbows, knees and bottom. Yellowish cholesterol deposits can also develop under the skin of the eyelids and the front surface of the eye (the cornea), leading to a grey-colored ring called an arcus cornealis.

You can find out if you have familial hypercholesterolemia with a DNA Test. If you have tested your blood levels of cholesterol and have a level above 300mg/dl, you may have FH.

How Are Fats Processed By The Body?

Let's take a look at the way our bodies process fats and saturated fats.

We know that genetically, some individuals may be more predisposed to higher levels of cholesterol. Familial hypercholesterolemia is a condition that affects up to 10% of the world's population. While FH only affects a relatively small number of the global population, there are a number of genes that can increase an individual's propensity to weight gain, high cholesterol and a higher risk of heart disease when consuming a diet that is high in saturated fat.

One of these is a variant known as the APOA5 gene. Certain variants of this genotype have been associated with higher fasting total cholesterol levels and LDL-cholesterol blood levels (which is sometimes known as our 'bad' cholesterol) plus lower HDL-cholesterol blood levels (which is sometimes known as our 'good' cholesterol). In individuals with this variant, the research indicates the benefits of eating a diet that is lower in fat with a reduced intake of omega-6 fats (these can be pro-inflammatory). More on this shortly.

Similarly individuals with a certain variant of the FABP2 gene may experience higher levels of LDL cholesterol and lower levels of HDL cholesterol and in these cases, lowering saturated fat intake and raising omega-3 intake can be helpful.

Our levels of HDL cholesterol also depend in part on the variant of the APOA2 gene we possess. This gene codes for Apolipoprotein A-II, a protein which is an important part of High-Density Lipoprotein (HDL) cholesterol. A certain variant in this gene has been associated with the reduced ability to produce Apolipoprotein A-II which has effects on saturated fat metabolism. Those with a certain variant of APOA2 are at increased risk of weight gain particularly visceral adipose tissue - the fat around the torso, if they consume a diet high in saturated fats. This can cause a significant amount of inflammation in the body which is linked to many chronic diseases from heart disease to cancer.

If you gain weight around your belly, look at the way your body processes fats. Also take a look at your stress levels and your sensitivity to sugars.

There are two other genes that I want to mention here which seem to impact the way some people gain fat more easily than others. Genetic obesity is closely associated with storage of fatty acids and the two of the most notable genes responsible for storing these fatty acids are the PPAR gene and the FTO gene.

Let's take a look at the PPAR gene.The Peroxisome proliferator-activated receptor gene is associated with weight gain when fat intake is high. The PPAR gamma gene is responsible for:

- the growth of new fat cells
- the storage of fatty acids
- the uptake of fatty acids.

A certain variant of the PPAR Gamma gene has shown significant increases in weight in response to dietary fat intake and monounsaturated fat intake - these include healthy fats like olive oil, avocados and certain types of nuts.

If you are thinking of going on the ketogenic diet or have been using it and are not seeing the results that you hoped for or you're putting on weight, it is worth checking your DNA to see what your genotype is.

In addition to this I would also suggest that you get some blood work done annually to check your triglyceride markers, including your triglycerides, your total cholesterol, your HDL, non-HDL and LDL cholesterol levels and your total cholesterol to HDL cholesterol ratio.

The other gene you may well have heard of is the FTO gene or Fat Mass and Obesity gene. Your genes are not your destiny and so if you have this gene do not despair. It does not mean that you will become obese or even fat. In fact I have two copies of the FTO gene and have never been fat. It's all about how your diet and lifestyle affect the expression of your genes.

However, the FTO gene does code for a protein associated with fat mass and obesity and it is responsible for regulating overall weight and bodyfat percentage. A high saturated fat intake is associated with FTO-induced weight gain and so if you have one or two copies of the FTO polymorphism, you are more likely to do better on a diet that is lower in saturated fat - particularly lower in things like butter, high fat dairy products, coconut oil and fatty cuts of meat such as beef, lamb or pork.

Those are some of the key genes that the scientific literature shows are implicated in the storage of fatty acids in your body - whether in the form of triglycerides in the blood or adipose tissue. The key takeaway here is that the way that your body processes fats, in part, comes down to your genetics. As such, before radically changing your diet it's worth testing your DNA and also getting some bloodwork done.

There are also genes that are implicated in the way that your body processes carbohydrates and your risk for metabolic diseases such as diabetes. If you are at higher risk for this then a ketogenic diet may well be a good option provided that you do not have the gene variants related to fatty acid metabolism that I have already mentioned.

What should you do if you have one or more of the genetic variants and fear the carbohydrates or can't thrive on something like the ketogenic diet? The answer may scare you a little! You may consider eating a higher carbohydrate diet that is high in fibre and lower in fat, keeping saturated fat intake to 7-10% of fats in your diet.

Consuming fats that are higher in unsaturated fats such as avocados and olive oil are safer than saturated fats that are commonly considered a healthy part of a keto diet. If you've been on a keto diet for a while then you may feel better increasing your carbohydrates slowly. The type of diet to follow would be one that is similar to that followed by the inhabitants of Kitava (a Blue Zone). A great book that you might want to read is 'The Blue Zones' by Dan Buettner. As previously mentioned, these areas across the world have the highest number of centenarians and are mostly free from chronic diseases like heart disease, cancer and diabetes. The Kitavans eat a diet which is rich in fibre dense carbohydrates such as starchy tubers, coconut meat and fresh fruit. They consume whole food sources of carbohydrates, not processed carbohydrates.

You can find out the exact type of diet that's right for you by testing your genetics with a DNA test (for more information on this go to www.rethinkhealth.club). The right DNA test will give you not just your sensitivity to fat and saturated fats but also your sensitivity to carbohydrates along with your omega-3 and 6 pathways and a whole host of other information.

Omega-3 and Omega-6 Pathways

Let's dive deeper into what omega-3 and omega-6 fats are. The human body is capable of producing all the fatty acids it needs, except for two: linoleic acid (LA) - an omega-6 fatty acid and alpha-linolenic acid (ALA) - an omega-3 fatty acid. Both of these fatty acids are needed for growth and repair but can also be used to make other fatty acids.

Your genetics can tell you a few things about the way that your body processes both omega-3 and omega-6 fatty acids.

Let's look at omega-3 first. Alpha-linolenic acid is a short chain omega-3 that is primarily found in plant based foods such as flaxseeds, walnuts and other nuts and seeds. Alpha-linolenic acid is an essential fatty acid because it cannot be produced in the body and so it has to be obtained through food.

People who follow a vegetarian or vegan diet and many other people, through choice, often prefer to consume plant sources of alpha-linolenic acid - things like flaxseeds and walnuts. The human body is not always able to effectively convert alpha-linolenic acid into the compounds that we need such as eicosapentaenoic acid (EPA) and docosahexaenoic acid (DHA). DHA and EPA are the critical fatty acids that can really help to enhance your performance and your brain health and they can also help in stabilizing ketosis. Animal sources are very bioavailable forms of DHA and EPA.

The scientific literature suggests that only between 2 and 10% of alpha-linolenic acid consumed is actually converted into DHA and EPA. When you're consuming DHA and EPA from animal sources it has the advantage that the animal has already done this for you. This is where we need to look at your FADS genes. The FADS1 gene relates to your omega-3 pathway.

Another gene to consider is known as the FADS2 Gene that encodes for activity in relation to omega-6 fats. In some individuals there is increased enzyme activity and that's been correlated with inflammatory states and a decreased need for omega-6. This is because the enzyme activity can impact downstream production of certain omega-6 fats which can lead to a heightened inflammatory state. In those individuals we would consider reducing omega-6 dietary sources and increasing omega-3s. In these individuals it would be particularly important to avoid processed vegetable oils and other processed omega-6 fats as these are likely to heighten the inflammatory state further.

The process of converting omega-6 fats into inflammatory compounds is called elongation. If you're somebody that has up-regulated elongation then a significant amount of the linoleic omega-6 fatty acid that you're consuming even from unprocessed food sources that are common on the keto diet, like cheese and nuts can get converted into arachidonic acid. Arachidonic acid is a precursor to inflammatory compounds.

If you fall within this category, to avoid higher levels of inflammation you need to avoid or reduce the common ketogenic fats sources that are high in linoleic acids - these are foods like eggs, nut butters and poultry. If you are consuming quite a large number of those foods then you should consider increasing your omega-3 fatty intake to offset this. The most bioavailable sources of omega-3 and particularly DHA and EPA are from smaller fish which are high in omega-3 and lower in toxins like mercury which travels up the food chain. An easy way to focus on the smaller, omega-3 rich fish sources is to use the acronym SMASH which stands for sardines, mackerel, anchovies, salmon and herrings.

All fats that you consume become incorporated into your cells - the membranes of cells are primarily formed from the fats that you eat. You want to ensure that you are not heating oils at excessively high temperatures. Even healthy oils such as extra virgin olive oil are unstable when heated too highly and can cause inflammation. Chronic inflammation can inhibit health and longevity.

The table below indicates the smoke point of various oils:

OIL / FAT	SMOKE POINT	BEST USES
Avocado Oil	520°F / 271°C	High heat cooking, low heat cooking, dressing, finishing
Ghee	480°F / 248°C	Baking, sauteing, high heat cooking
Coconut Oil	450°F / 232°C	Baking, sauteing, high heat cooking
Peanut Oil	450°F / 232°C	High heat cooking
Sesame Oil	450°F / 232°C	Dressing, finishing
Rice Bran Oil	415°F / 212°C	Medium-heat cooking
Macadamia Nut Oil	410°F / 210°C	Medium-heat cooking, dressing, finishing
Olive Oil	410°F / 210°C	Medium heat cooking, dressing, finishing
Tallow (Beef Fat)	400°F / 204°C	Medium heat cooking
Walnut Oil	400°F / 204°C	Dressing, finishing
Duck Fat	375°F / 190°C	Medium-heat cooking
Lard (Pork Fat)	375°F / 190°C	Medium-heat cooking
Butter	300°F / 140°C	Low-heat cooking, finishing
Flaxseed Oil	225°F / 107°C	Dressing, finishing

This is also where doing some blood work can be important, particularly if your DNA test has identified that these pathways may be impaired. Your DNA can give you details of your pathways and risk factors and your blood work will show you what your current omega-3 to omega-6 ratios are. Ideally you would want to be aiming for an omega-6 to omega-3 ratio of no higher than 3:1. In a typical American diet this ratio can be as high as 16:1. This is definitely something worth looking at both from a genetic perspective and then also checking your blood work routinely - I would suggest annually.

The scientific literature seems to indicate that the ability to convert omega-3 into DHA and EPA is in part due to ancestry with ALA conversion being better amongst African, Indian, Pakistani, Bangladeshi and Sri Lankan populations. It seems less common in Europeans and Native Americans, although there is variation depending on which part of Europe you originate from. Individuals from the northern hemisphere are often less able to convert ALA into DHA and EPA. This seems at least in part, to be down to where the ancestral populations lived over time. In far Northern European, Native American, Iberian or indigneous Arctic populations they would likely have consumed DHA and EPA directly through animal and fish sources. It's worth finding out with a DNA test what type of variant you have because then you can target your omega-3 intake and in particular your DHA and EPA intake to keep inflammation low and optimise your health.

DETOXIFICATION

Your DNA can also give you other important information to dive deeper into areas of your body that actually need support. One of the key areas that we would look at in this regard is your detoxification pathways primarily looking at both phase 1 and phase 2 detoxification.

In relation to phase 1 detoxification what we are looking at here primarily is the cooking of certain meat products at high temperatures. When you cook meat at high temperatures it accelerates the formation of chemicals that are not actually naturally present in uncooked meat. Some of these chemicals (known as heterocyclic amines and polycyclic aromatic hydrocarbons) are regarded as toxic compounds and can actually damage the DNA and protein in the cells leading to some pretty serious health problems in the long run.

Meat or fish that is cooked at very high temperatures or for a very long time, creates the highest levels of these chemicals. Avoid or limit (to maximum 1-2 weekly) char-grilled meat or smoked meat or fish particularly if your phase 1 detoxification operates at a faster rate. In people with faster phase 1 detoxification it can lead to these chemicals being metabolized more quickly and possibly overwhelming your body's system.

If you do have a faster processing speed, the advice is to limit your intake of char grilled or smoked meat or fish or things like blackened chicken and barbecued meats to no more than once per week. This is where including some cruciferous vegetables alongside the meal can enhance the detoxification process as they contain lots of beneficial anti-cancer compounds. This is definitely an area to be aware of, particularly if you're consuming quite a lot of meat in your diet on something like the carnivore diet.

In relation to phase 2 detoxification, GST enzymes relate to the production of glutathione. In particular there are two genes that have been well studied - GSTM1 and GSTT1. These are either going to be present or deleted, and again a DNA test will indicate if one or more of these are deleted.

If you have one or more deletions you are likely to be at an increased risk of oxidative stress, inflammation and carcinogenesis so you might be someone who would have more difficulty processing the compounds that can be produced from meat cooked at high temperatures. This can also affect your processing of excess hormones (like estrogen) and that's why it's really important to make sure that your liver function is optimal and that inflammation is low.

These GST enzymes are induced by certain compounds that you can get from your diet so if you have got a deletion of one of these genes, for example, then you would want to make sure that you're increasing your consumption of cruciferous vegetables. Cruciferous vegetables include broccoli, broccoli sprouts and cauliflower. These vegetables contain glucosinolates which can be very helpful in activating the GST enzymes. Curcumin from turmeric is also good. Bear in mind that turmeric in itself is actually not that bioavailable unless it's combined with something like black pepper or some fats to enhance its absorption. This is where taking a good quality curcumin supplement can be helpful. The other food I suggest increasing (unless you have sensitivities to them) would be the allium family of vegetables - onions, leeks and scallions.

ANTIOXIDANTS, B VITAMINS AND VITAMIN D

Uncovering your DNA results can also tell you about your vitamin and antioxidant needs to help you optimise your health further. You can gain an understanding of your vitamin needs including vitamin D and also your antioxidant needs.

Vitamin D

Looking first at vitamin D, what we see is that in some individuals their vitamin D receptor gene functions less well. In those individuals even when they are exposed to sunlight (which is our main way of synthesising vitamin D) they tend not to synthesise it terribly well.

Many people are not getting enough vitamin D especially during the winter months and according to the British Medical Journal, vitamin D deficiency is the most under diagnosed medical condition in both children and adults. This is generally because patients don't typically present with clinical signs until the deficiency is pretty severe and prolonged and includes issues like rickets developing in children. In adults they may experience bone pain and muscle weakness.

There are lots of people with undiagnosed vitamin D deficiency. In addition to the skeletal effects, it is now recognised that vitamin D deficiency increases the risk of many chronic diseases, including cancer, autoimmune diseases, type 2 diabetes, heart disease and hypertension, neurocognitive dysfunction such as dementia, infectious diseases (including upper respiratory tract infections), osteoarthritis, as well as depression and schizophrenia.

So how do we get vitamin D? Vitamin D is formed when sunlight converts a cholesterol molecule known as 7-dehydrocholesterol into an active form of vitamin D.

Vitamin D travels through your blood and tissues like a kind of wifi signal and enters into your cells. Once inside, it binds to a receptor molecule called the vitamin D receptor gene which allows the vitamin D to enter into the cell nucleus (where your DNA is housed) and switches on over 900 genes.

The activity of these genes affect a wide range of processes including bone formation and metabolism, lowering of inflammation and the suppressing of tumour formation. Some are also responsible for creating and maintaining brain synapses. As such,vitamin D is important for your neurological health too.

Essentially when vitamin D is too low, the right genes are not activated.

How can you know whether or not you should be supplementing with vitamin D?

Firstly, you should get your serum vitamin D checked at least annually, especially if you live in a country in the Northern hemisphere.

Vitamin D serum tests usually check the inactive form - 25-hydroxycholecalciferol. You want your levels of this to be between 50 to 80ng/ml.

The 100x Rule

Once you have your serum levels, you can work out how much vitamin D you need to take as a supplement, if any. To do this you use the 100X rule. You subtract your serum vitamin D level from your goal, e.g. 80 and multiply the difference by 100 to get the dose in IUs. So if your current Vitamin D is 30ng/ml and you want to achieve a level of 80ng/ml, you would take 5,000 IUs = (80-30) x 100. Always check blood serum levels first and regularly during treatment and work with a qualified health practitioner.

Ideally, look for a vitamin D3 supplement with K2. The K2 helps to ensure that calcium is absorbed easily and reaches the bone mass, while preventing arterial calcification. This helps to keep your heart and bones healthy. Separately, K2 regulates normal blood clotting.

You probably don't need to take vitamin D in summer if you are spending enough time outdoors (without sunscreen) or are going on a holiday somewhere hot. Fortunately, you cannot overdose on vitamin D from the sun as your body will simply stop making it. However, you do need to take care with sun exposure as this can cause skin cancer.

Energy and B Vitamins

Another area that your DNA test can really help with is giving you your B vitamin needs and how well your body functions in terms of a process known as methylation. I'm looking here specifically at the methylation genes and in particular the MTHFR Gene. This can be impaired by up to 70% in some individuals and in those individuals it's important that you make sure that you're including enough sources of vitamin B6, B12 and B9 in your diet. Ideally you would want to get as many of these as possible from your food, but if you have gut health problems, your blood results show you need supplementation or you want to boost levels, a good quality B complex can help. When supplementing with folic acid, you want to make sure that you're using a natural form of folate as opposed to folic acid which is the synthetic form.

If your genetic test indicates that you may need support with methylation, I would recommend that you follow up with a homocysteine blood test. A high level of homocysteine is a risk factor for cardiovascular disease and so it's a good indicator of how effectively the body is methylating. If your homocysteine seems high then you can take steps working with a functional medicine practitioner to lower your homocysteine levels. It may also be worth looking at the wider methylation cycle in terms of functional testing.

Antioxidants

The other point I'd like to come onto regarding DNA for health optimisation, is that it can also indicate your antioxidant needs. The human body creates much of the antioxidants it needs itself including in the form of superoxide dismutase, catalase and glutathione. If you have a raised antioxidant need then it can be really important to try to get as many antioxidants as you can from dietary sources as well as including compounds that support your antioxidant status like lycopene, resveratrol and glutathione (more on this and sirtuin-activating compounds below).

Including plenty of herbs and spices in your diet can help with this too, as can foods that are dark in colour, such as berries and dark chocolate.

Food Allergies & Intolerances

Many people tend to talk about DNA testing for food intolerances. This isn't really the best way to discover food intolerances. It can give you a limited amount of information in a couple of areas, relating to lactose tolerance and your predisposition to celiac disease.

What we do know is that not all people are able to produce the enzyme lactase after the age of three years old. Lactase is what you need to digest lactose which is a sugar contained in milk and some other dairy products. The literature indicates that a large percentage of the world's population are actually not able to digest lactose after the age of around 3 years old. Up until the age of 3 years old most people can digest it because lactose is contained in breast milk, but after that we may not have genes that dictate lactase persistence. A DNA test can be really useful in finding out whether you are lactose intolerant.

You can also discover some information around your gluten sensitivity so you can find out whether you're at a higher risk for gluten intolerance and celiac disease. While not a conclusive answer, it can help point you in the right direction of doing an elimination diet or even doing some functional tests to establish whether you do have either celiac disease or non-celiac gluten sensitivity.

There is more information coming out about DNA testing all the time.

Certain DNA testing companies can test your risk factors for certain types of cancer. You can also test for your responses to certain drugs and the way in which we process those drugs.

Food allergies are different to food intolerances with the latter not necessarily showing immediately after a food is eaten. If you experience gas, bloating, unpredictable bowel movements, skin issues such as rosacea or eczema, you may be intolerant to certain types of foods. It is worth finding out about these either through an elimination diet or through high sensitivity testing to uncover if you have any food intolerances. If you continue to eat food(s) that you are intolerant to, it can increase inflammation in the body and also irritate the lining of the gut, potentially leading to issues such as leaky gut.

GUT HEALTH

Another area to look at when designing your diet is your microbiome. This is an important and emerging area at the time of writing.

Getting your microbiome tested enables you to better understand the levels of both healthy and potentially harmful bacteria in your gut and also to determine whether or not inflammation is present. Understanding your microbiome and balance of gut bacteria can also give you information on the way that you process certain foods.

The volume of DNA in our microbiome far exceeds the amount of human DNA. Some gut tests analyse the types of bacteria present in your gut in proportion to the overall microbiome. It gives you information about the various functions of the bacteria that are residing in your gut, what vitamins they synthesise and to a certain extent, the degree to which they protect you against certain diseases and inflammation. You can get specific recommendations to improve and maintain the balance of your microbiome. The data on this is emerging as it is a new and developing area. Some of these tests are consumer tests which can be done yourself, while others such as the comprehensive tests from laboratories such as Genova Diagnostics usually require working with a functional medical doctor or nutritional practitioner.

YOUR GUT IS YOUR GARDEN

Testing aside, there are a number of things that you can include in your diet to help protect the health of your gut.

Think of your gut as your garden. If you want it to flourish with with beneficial bacteria that among other things, help you digest your food, absorb vitamins, lower your risk of obesity, enhance your immune system and lower your risk of depression (up to 90% of serotonin is made in the gut), then you want to look after this garden of beautiful plants (beneficial bacteria), keep the weeds to a minimum (the harmful bacteria) and keep its borders strong (your gut lining).

How can you do this? Firstly as mentioned above, avoid foods that you are intolerant to and which irritate the lining of the gut. Secondly, include plenty of foods that help to plant and encourage the growth of beneficial bacteria.

These include[32]:

- fermented foods such as sauerkraut, pickles and kimchi
- live yoghurt - Greek-style or coconut
- kefir - fermented milk with good bacteria
- miso - fermented soy beans with healthy bacteria and enzymes
- sourdough - if you're going to eat bread, this is the bread to eat as the dough is fermented and more easily digestible

If you have irritation with your gut lining or inflammation, taking a supplement such as colostrum, bone broth or glutamine can help. You should aim to the bottom of what is causing problems with your gut and working with a good functional medicine practitioner or functional nutritionist can help.

EAT SIRTUIN ACTIVATING COMPOUNDS (STACs)

When structuring your personalised nutrition plan, many people are not aware of the enormous benefits of including foods that activate an ancient family of genes, known as sirtuins.

What are Sirtuins?

Sirtuins are regulators of cellular health and metabolism. They were first discovered in yeast in 1984.

Dr Amar Klar, a geneticist, discovered the first sirtuin (SIRT2) in the 1970s identifying it as a gene that controlled the ability of yeast cells to

32 be careful with these if you have a difficulty with histamine tolerance

mate. In the 1990s, researchers found the genes that were similar in structure to SIRT2 in other organisms including fruit flies and worms. They renamed these sirtuins and found that different organisms had differing numbers of sirtuins, with humans and mice each having seven sirtuins, yeast having five and bacteria having one.

In humans, these sirtuins play a role in aging and metabolic health. In 1991, MIT biologist Leonard Guarante, alongside graduate students Nick Austriaco and Brian Kennedy, conducted experiments to understand how yeast aged. He identified SIRT2 as a gene that promoted longevity in yeast. Research is continuing as to how SIRT2 might affect longevity in humans.

Sirtuins have been shown to remove acetyl groups from proteins. Acetyl groups are tags on proteins that are recognised by other proteins that interact with the acetyl tags.

To understand what acetylation is and why it's important, we need to go back to what you learnt about DNA . DNA is wrapped around large proteins known as histones into a condensed form called chromatin.

DNA is packed into chromosomes in the form of chromatin. Chromatin is made up of DNA, histone proteins and non-histone proteins.

For our DNA to be activated and transcribed in real time, the chromatin needs to be uncoiled so that it can be read. This process is known as acetylation. Deacetylation is the opposite - it involves removing acetyl groups so that the chromatin has less transcription and is coiled back up. Why is this important? It is important because it is effectively silencing genes. This is key to health and longevity because if DNA stays unwound, it is more vulnerable to damage.

So how does it get deacetylated? This is through the sirtuin family of genes. As already mentioned, in humans there are 7 sirtuins and SIRT2 is the one that has been most studied in relation to the ability to prolong life.

What's really important here is that SIRT2 is only able to deacetylate in the presence of a coenzyme called nicotinamide adenine dinucleotide (NAD+).

According to David Sinclair, a professor in the Department of Genetics, co-director of the Paul F. Glenn Center for the Biology of Aging at Harvard Medical School and author of the book 'Lifespan', the key compound that enhances the activity of all seven sirtuins is NAD+. NAD+ is produced in the body but declines with age.

NAD AND THE POWER TO AGE BACKWARDS

NAD is a powerful anti-aging molecule and a coenzyme. Coenzymes are compounds that certain enzymes need to perform basic functions and keep you alive. Without NAD+, as David Sinclair writes in his book, 'Lifespan', you would be dead within 60 seconds. NAD+ is required for a number of processes in the body including:

- creating energy in the mitochondria (the "powerhouses" of your cells)
- sending messages between nerve cells
- maintaining blood glucose levels at night
- proper muscle contractions
- generating ketones.

NAD is like a delivery guy picking up an electron from one location (when it becomes NADH) and then dropping it off at another location (where it becomes NAD+ again).

NAD levels naturally decline with age. By the time a person is aged fifty, levels of NAD+ have fallen to half of their youthful levels. This results in a loss in both sirtuin and PARP activity (more on PARP later).

Studies in mice have shown that treating old mice with PARP inhibitors or precursors to NAD+ can greatly improve insulin sensitivity, reverse mitochondrial dysfunction, reduce stem cell senescence (when cells stop dividing, typically in response to DNA damage) and extend lifespan.

There are various practices you can engage in to enhance levels of NAD+ naturally:

- Practice intermittent fasting and/or caloric restriction

- Follow a cyclical ketogenic diet. Ketones have been shown to increase the ratio of NAD+ to NADH. Your body produces ketones naturally when you are fasting for 12 hours or more, restricting carbohydrates, taking exogenous ketones or using MCT oil (preferably including pure caprylic acid or C8).

Certain supplements can also enhance the production of NAD+. One way to enhance the production of NAD+ is to take NMN - β-Nicotinamide Mononucleotide or NR - Nicotanimide Riboside. NR is converted to NMN and so some people take NR as it is cheaper to buy than NMN. Niacin and Nicotinamide are even cheaper, but according to Dr Sinclair, they do not seem to raise NAD levels in the way that NR and NMN do.

Raising NAD+ helps to enhance sirtuin activity.

GET YOUR STACs

There are incredible benefits that you can get by including sirtuin-activating compounds (STACs) in your diet.

STACs activate the sirtuin genes in the same way that caloric restriction, intermittent fasting and exercise do. What that means is that these powerful foods mimic the effects of fasting and exercise. They can be a very powerful addition and help you to live healthier, leaner and longer.

The gene that has been well studied for driving fat loss is Sirt-1. In studies in mice, mice that have been genetically engineered to have high levels of Sirt-1 are leaner and more metabolically active with mice that lack Sirt-1 being fatter with greater incidence of metabolic disease.[33]

In human studies, it has been shown that obese individuals have lower levels of Sirt-1 in their bodyfat[34]. In another study, it was shown that people who are leaner and less likely to struggle with weight gain have higher levels of Sirt-1 gene activity.[35]

Consuming foods that are rich in sirtuin-activating compounds (STACs) enhances the activity of sirtuins. The other great thing about foods rich in sirtuins is that they are master regulators or our metabolism. So not only can they help you live younger for longer, they can also help you to stay lean and fit. Aiden Goggins and Glen Matten talk about this in their great book "The Sirtfood Diet: The Original and Official Sirtfood Diet That's Taken the Celebrity World by Storm". As the authors elaborate, foods rich in sirtuin-activating

33 Chalkiadaki, A. & Guarente, L. "High-fat diet triggers inflammation-induced cleavage of SIRT1 in adipose tissue to promote metabolic dysfunction - https://www.ncbi.nlm.nih.gov/pubmed/22883230

34 SIRT1 transcription is decreased in visceral adipose tissue of morbidly obese patients with severe hepatic steatosis https://www.ncbi.nlm.nih.gov/pubmed/20033348

35 SIRT1 genetic variation is related to BMI and risk of obesity - https://www.ncbi.nlm.nih.gov/pubmed/19741164

compounds (STACS), have a significant impact on fat burning while also increasing muscle and enhancing cellular fitness.

Consuming sirtuin rich foods and taking sirtuin activators may be a powerful combination for enhancing metabolism, reducing cellular damage and enhancing youthfulness. Sirtuins help to protect your cells from oxidative stress and the resulting decline. They help your body repair DNA that has been damaged from everyday functions and exposure to toxins. Sirtuins also play a role in helping to maintain the length of your telomeres (more on this later).

What are the foods that contain the highest number of sirtuin-activating compounds (STACs)? These include:

- Apples
- Bird's Eye Chilli
- Blueberries
- Broccoli
- Cacao and cacao nibs
- Capers
- Celery (including leaves)
- Cucumbers
- Dark leafy vegetables
- Extra virgin olive oil
- Grapes
- Green tea (higher in Matcha green tea)
- Kale
- Parsley
- Peppers
- Pomegranate
- Red onion
- Organic red wine (especially pinot noir and if dry farmed)
- Rocket

- Strawberries
- Turmeric
- Walnuts

The Energiser Juice (sirtuin booster):

1 green apple

½ head of celery

2 inch chunk of ginger (optional)*

1 handful of flat leaf parsley

½ large cucumber

Juice of 1 lime

Juice all of the ingredients together and pour over ice. Drink on an empty stomach 15-30 minutes before food.

EZ WATER

Celery Juice and other vegetable juices provide a rich source of exclusion zone water ("EZ water"). This is the fourth phase of water discovered by Dr Gerald Pollack. EZ water or structured water, is viscous like honey - in between solid and liquid in consistency. Your cells use EZ water and it delivers electrons to your mitochondria - the powerhouses of your cells. This helps the mitochondria to generate more energy.

You can also make EZ water by shaking or blending water. Water absorbs vibrational energy when you blend it. It has been shown to form more easily when there are small droplets of fat present and this is because the fat helps to create a piezoelectric effect. As Dave Asprey notes in his book 'Headstrong', the act of blending fat and water together creates more EZ water. One way to do this in a polyphenol rich beverage is to make bulletproof coffee.

As Dave Asprey explains in another one of his books, 'Superhuman', when he was in the Tibetan mountains he noticed that the locals always carried blenders with portable batteries to make their yak butter tea. Both tea and coffee contain large amounts of polyphenols. Coffee contains both melanin and melanoidins which are created during the coffee roasting process. During the roasting process, coffee beans undergo structural changes that lead to the formation of melanoidins. Melanoidins are high molecular weight nitrogenous and brown-colored compounds. Several biological activities, including antioxidant, antimicrobial, anticarcinogenic, anti-inflammatory, antihypertensive, and antiglycative activities have been attributed to coffee melanoidins.[36]

Dave Asprey considers that one of the main reasons that Bulletproof Coffee and Yak butter tea are so energising is because

36 Food & Function: Coffee melanoidins: structures, mechanisms of formation and potential health impacts https://doi.org/10.1039/C2FO30048F

the mechanical vibrations from the blender break up the melanin and the melanoidins giving your mitochondria free oxygen and electrons to use for energy.

Here's my own favourite bulletproof coffee recipe with a twist:

1 shot espresso

100ml water

½ - 1 tbsp raw cacao butter

1tsp MCT oil

1 tsp maca powder

SHOULD YOU BUY ORGANIC?

A common and legitimate question asked by many is should I buy organic and is it worth the extra price? While studies of the nutrient content in organic foods vary in results and nutrient content seems to vary from farmer to farmer and year to year, reviews of multiple studies do show that organic varieties provide significantly greater levels of certain vitamins and minerals than non-organic varieties. This includes greater levels of vitamin C, iron, magnesium and phosphorus. Organic foods have also been shown to be significantly lower in levels of nitrates and pesticides.

Organic foods also typically provide higher levels of antioxidant phytochemicals - flavonoids, anthocyanins and carotenoids.[37]

37 https://pubmed.ncbi.nlm.nih.gov/20359265/

HORMESIS AND XENOHORMESIS (THE BENEFITS OF STRESSED PLANTS)

There are two powerful concepts that have emerged in recent years that may help to both enhance our health and longevity. These are hormesis and xenohormesis.

To understand this we need to look first at the concept of the adaptive stress response. One of the fundamental processes of life is the ability of organisms to respond to physical, chemical and social stressors.[38]

Hormesis is the concept that low levels of stress can improve the health, adaptability, fitness and well-being of an organism's health through the stimulation of the cellular stress response.[39] Examples of this would be a strength based workout where the stimulation and breakdown of muscle fibres causes a stress response that enables the body to become stronger. For hormesis to be effective in causing adaptation, the dose needs to be correct. In other words you can have too much stimulation which actually results in a potential weakening of the response. More on this in Chapter 5.

A second concept is that of interconnectedness of different living organisms on the planet. This brings me onto the concept of xenohormesis which is the process by which one organism benefits from the stress response of another. [40]

An example of this is how a stressed plant is able to confer that stress tolerance to the animals or humans that consume them. Since plants cannot physically move away from stresses such as

38 (Feder and Hofmann 1999; Selye 1978; Tytell and Hooper 2001; Welch 1993).

39 (Calabrese and Baldwin 2003; Gerber et al. 1999; Rattan 2008)

40 (Howitz et al. 2003; Howitz and Sinclair 2008)

a lack of water nutrient availability or extremes of temperature and environmental factors, these have to be endured in place. This stimulates a stress response in the plant and this has been evolving in plants for almost 1 billion years.

Plants that are grown under less than ideal conditions, ones that do not maximise the crop yield, may offer more beneficial nutrients than those that are grown in conditions to maximise crop yield, as is the case in mono-crop farming.

An example of this is in the production of wine. The grapes that confer the most health benefits and often taste better are those grown in relatively dry sun exposed in fertile soil. Wines grown in this way are often shown to have higher levels of resveratrol which protects the plant by reducing damage from UV and also eliminating pathogenic moulds. Resveratrol has been shown to activate the mammalian stress response system and to extend longevity.

Another example is in the case of strawberries and blueberries. Wild strawberries and blueberries grown in drought-stress conditions have higher antioxidant levels, phenol content and also taste better than those that are cultivated in more controlled conditions.

Polyphenols and phenols

The beneficial compounds polyphenols and phenols can be divided into flavonoids and non flavonoids. Flavonoids include:

- Rutin
- Quercetin
- Epigallocatechin gallate (EGCG)
- Isoflavones
- Anthocyanins.

Non-flavonoids include:

- Hydroxybenzoic acid
- Stilbene derivatives such as resveratrol, curcumin, cinnamic acid, caffeic acid, rosmarinic acid and ferulic acid.[41]

Xeno-hormetic plant compounds can benefit the animal human eating them in two main ways - either directly or by activating the consumers own stress defence pathways. In some cases such as for vitamins C and E, the compounds act as antioxidants whereas in other cases with polyphenols such as resveratrol and curcumin, they stimulate the animal stress response. These bioactive plant compounds may improve longevity in humans and animals by activating or priming their cellular survival pathways. These compounds are classified as 'caloric restriction mimetics' as they activate the stress response in a similar way to caloric deprivation or fasting.

By engaging in monocrop farming we may be losing important nutritional and health benefits that are conferred when we consume agricultural products that have been subjected to the stress that exist in more natural environments.

Some of the compounds that you may wish to include in your diet to promote longevity and benefit from xenohormesis are the following:

Curcumin

Curcumin is a compound produced by some plants and probably best known to be obtained from turmeric (curcuma longa). Curcumin is a powerful antioxidant and anti-inflammatory that works in a few different ways. It is a potent antioxidant, protecting cells from reactive oxygen species. It also enhances your body's own natural antioxidant capacity by improving the production of certain antioxidant enzymes such as glutathione, catalase and

41 https://www.ncbi.nlm.nih.gov/pmc/articles/PMC3024065/#:~:text=Xenohormesis%20is%20a%20biological%20principle,to%20animals%20that%20consume%20them.

superoxide dismutase. As you may remember when we looked at DNA and raised antioxidant needs, some individuals produce lower levels of these endogenous antioxidants and so consuming curcumin may help to support this. In this way curcumin can also help to reduce chronic inflammation throughout the body. Curcumin has low bioavailability and also constitutes only 3 to 5% of the turmeric root. It is therefore difficult to get enough curcumin by simply consuming turmeric. If you're using turmeric in cooking, combining it with black pepper or piperine (a black pepper extract) or with a high-quality fat source such as olive oil, coconut oil or grass fed butter can help to improve the bioavailability. If you want to get the benefits of curcumin it may be better to consume it as a supplement rather than simply through food.

Pterostilbene

Pterostilbene is a derivative of the antioxidant phenyl resveratrol. It is structurally very similar to resveratrol but may be better absorbed and potentially a more potent antioxidant and anti-cancer molecule. Pterostilbene can be found in blueberries and is also a compound that can be taken in supplement form. The benefits of it are wide-ranging and seem to include reducing glucose and cholesterol in animals. It exhibits strong anti-inflammatory capabilities and may also increase levels of NAD.

Coenzyme Q10 (CoQ10)

Coenzyme Q10 (CoQ10) is a natural compound found in mammals and is a powerful anti-aging tool. CoQ10 is an essential component in the mitochondrial electron transport chain and is an antioxidant that is found in lipoproteins and plasma membranes throughout the body.

The synthesis of CoQ10 tends to decline with age and so as you get older, supplementing with it may be very beneficial. CoQ10 is also found in organic meats and oily fish such as salmon.

Glutathione

Glutathione is an antioxidant that is naturally produced by the body, commonly referred to as the 'master antioxidant'. It supports whole body detoxification, helping cells grow, multiply and repair themselves. As glutathione has a wide-ranging antioxidant activity in the body it plays a role in aging. As we age, we tend to see a decrease in glutathione levels and this seems to affect the onset of some chronic diseases. There are three main ways that you can support glutathione in the body. The first is by supporting your body's own natural production of glutathione through consumption of the following foods:

- Selenium rich foods such as chicken, fish, beef, cottage cheese and brown rice
- Foods high in vitamin C such as strawberries, blackcurrants, broccoli, red peppers and oranges
- Turmeric - curcumin in turmeric helps to enhance glutathione levels and improve glutathione activity
- Essential amino acids or whey protein - the amino acids glutamine, cysteine and glycine are used for glutathione synthesis.

You can also consume foods that are naturally higher in glutathione. These include steak, chicken, pork loin, asparagus, avocadoes, broccoli, spinach, parsley and tomatoes.

Finally you can take a glutathione supplement. Sublingual supplements (taken under the tongue) may be better absorbed as they bypass digestion. Another more effective form are liposomal supplements - the liposomes (tiny fat droplets) protect the glutathione until the liposomes are taken up by your cells and broken down releasing the glutathione.

Glutathione supplements can be expensive and so an alternative is to take N-acetyl L-cysteine (NAC) which is a glutathione precursor. This has been used in therapeutic practices for several decades may help to replenish intracellular glutathione.

Quercetin

Quercetin is a flavonoid that is naturally found in green tea, apples, ginkgo biloba, red wine and white wine. Levels of quercetin are actually higher in white wine than in red wine. It also occurs in naturally high concentrations in yellow chilli peppers, onions and capers. Quercetin is a powerful antioxidant and research indicates that it may be one of the most powerful flavonoids for combating free radicals. This effect does seem to be dose-dependent as high concentrations may cause quercetin to become a reactive oxygen species in itself. Quercetin enhances your body's own antioxidant producing abilities and has been shown to improve the endogenous production by the body of superoxide dismutase, catalase and glutathione.

Pyrroloquinoline Quinone (PQQ)

Pyrroloquinoline Quinone (PQQ) is an antioxidant with over 175 published studies to show its wide-ranging benefits for improving general cognition, mood, mental processing power and memory. PQQ has also been shown to increase mitochondrial density, reduce inflammation and defend against oxidative stress. It is naturally found in celery, papaya, kiwi, sweet potatoes, parsley, green tea and fermented bean products like natto.

You can also take PQQ in supplement form and when used in combination with CoQ10 they seem to synergistically increase their potency. Ideally look for a form called BioPQQ as it is formulated from natural bacterial fermentation rather than synthetic form.

Sulforaphane

Sulforaphane is a sulphur based molecule that is naturally found in cruciferous vegetables like broccoli, kale, cauliflower, cabbage, radishes, mustard greens and brussel sprouts. Research suggests that it is effective at activating your body's own antioxidant producing processes. It has also been shown to induce autophagy (cellular recycling and death) and also stimulates the production of more mitochondria helping to enhance energy.

Sulforaphane is formed when you chew raw cruciferous vegetables. Essentially chewing with our teeth breaks apart the plant cell walls. This causes a chemical called glucoraphanin to combine with another chemical called myrosinase. When these two chemicals combine they create a new compound - sulforaphane. Sulforaphane is toxic to insects but elicits a defence response in humans and activates enzymes that help you to neutralise and excrete environmental toxins. It is a powerful tool in aiding detoxification.

Be aware that cooking inactivates myrosinase which is needed to create sulforaphane. Certain types of gut bacteria can convert some of the remaining glucoraphanin into sulforaphane but you can also use a pretty punchy and effective hack to enhance sulforaphane production. After cooking your cruciferous vegetables add half a teaspoon of mustard seed powder. By adding the mustard seed powder you will regain the ability to create sulforaphane. It also tastes pretty good!

Broccoli sprouts are also a good addition to your diet as they contain up to 100 times the sulforaphane producing capacity of adult broccoli.

Cruciferous vegetables also contain other compounds that aid in detoxification including cyano hydroxy butane and diindoyl-methane (DIM). You can also take DIM in supplement form which can be particularly helpful in treating and preventing acne.

Epigallocatechin Gallate (EGCG)

Epigallocatechin Gallate (EGCG) is the primary molecule contained in green tea that acts as a free radical scavenger and also activates the body's own antioxidant production. Research indicates that EGCG is more potent than vitamin C and vitamin E. EGCG also promotes cellular autophagy and certain cells including those in the liver and it may also improve weight loss by increasing fat oxidation. EGCG easily crosses the blood-brain barrier and may be neuroprotective, reducing inflammation in the brain. It can also be taken in supplement form.

Omega-3 oils

You may recall from earlier the importance of getting the optimal ratio of omega-6 to omega-3 and also the anti-inflammatory properties of DHA and EPA and the cognitive and physical benefits of these.

More and more studies are emerging on the benefits of fish oil and new research indicates that it may be effective at staving off cardiovascular and metabolic issues that can occur with aging such as diabetes.Micronutrients in fish oil such as omega-3 fatty acids and also notably vitamin D, have also been shown to have an impact on telomere length (an indicator of biological aging, more on this below).

Supplementing with fish oil at a dose of 2.5 grams per day has been shown to lead to a 32% reduction in telomere shortening.

In studies with middle-aged rats, fish oil has also been shown to increase the activities of the antioxidants glutathione superoxide dismutase and catalase as well as total antioxidant capacity. I personally take between 2 and 4 grams of fish oil daily. When taking fish oil in supplement form, it is important to make sure that you take a pure fish oil that has not been oxidised and contains an antioxidant like vitamin E alongside it to prevent oxidation, otherwise it may cause more harm than good.

TELOMERES

Telomeres are the caps on the chromosomes in your cells that help to protect them from damage. Over time and as we age, through repeated cell division, inflammation and oxidative stress, telomeres wear out and shorten. This eventually leaves your cells' chromosomes unprotected and the wear and tear begins to affect your DNA. You can think of telomeres as similar to the caps on the end of shoelaces that keep the shoelaces from fraying. Their job is to protect the chromosomes from being damaged or tangling with each other, but over time they get shorter until eventually they may disappear.

Telomerase is an enzyme that lengthens telomeres and stops them from wearing out too fast or too early.

The amount of telomerase produced by the body can be detrimentally affected by chronic stress, lack of exercise, low plant consumption, and a lack of stress reducing practices such as mindfulness, meditation and yoga. At the time of writing, the best known way to maximize the longevity enhancing effects of telomerase is to switch on the gene that is responsible for producing it.

If you are practising the principles contained in the previous and following chapters of this book then you will be going a long way towards helping maintain your telomere length. Pay particular attention to the stress reducing practices contained in Chapter 5.

Astragalus can also help to enhance telomere length. Astragalus is a herb that comes from the root of a perennial plant that grows in Northern and Eastern China. Astragalus extract needs to be taken in very high doses to provide benefit to activating telomerase. The adaptogenic herb complex TianChi contains high amounts of astragalus in a pure concentrated extraction. Astragalus has also been used in traditional Chinese medicine as a tonic and is said to build upright Chi, promoting good posture.

There are other herbs that may increase telomerase production and these include bacopa monnieri, boswellia, ashwagandha, green tea and milk thistle. Omega-3 fatty acids from fish oil, curcumin, resveratrol and the amino acid L-carnitine may also help the body to produce telomerase. More recently, certain varieties of mushrooms such as reishi, cordyceps, oyster, shiitake and wood ear have been studied for their ability to increase telomerase activity.

MEASURING YOUR BIOLOGICAL AGE

In recent times, laboratories have developed the technology to measure the rate at which your telomeres shorten. At home testing companies use varying technologies, including analyzing DNA methylation patterns to measure biological aging. This method is based on Dr. Steve Horvath's epigenetic aging clock which has been cited in over 600 peer reviewed scientific publications.

Companies such as Chronomics look at epigenetics to reveal how a person's health is being shaped by lifestyle and environment over time. Epigenetic information decides which genes are turned 'on' or 'off' and this ultimately affects the risk of developing chronic illnesses (such as different types of cancer, type 2 diabetes, cardiovascular disease or neurodegenerative diseases).

The Chronomics test enables you to measure how specific interventions (for instance changes in diet, exercise or sleep) are affecting your molecular health so that you can help change nutritional and lifestyle strategies for the better.

FOODS AND COMPOUNDS TO SUPPORT A HEALTHY BRAIN

Some of the compounds that I have mentioned above that are associated with enhancing longevity are also often included in a range of supplements that are known as nootropics.

To ensure healthy brain function and cognition, we first need to avoid unhealthy eating patterns and consuming certain foods that can harm our brains including:

- Highly processed foods (especially those that contain processed vegetable oils),
- Foods that are high in heavy metals such as mercury (e.g. from large fish like swordfish),
- Artificially sweetened foods
- Hydrogenated fats
- Gluten (which as been associated autoimmune diseases, neuroinflammation and gut damage)[42]
- Foods that contain mycotoxins (mould) that are commonly found in foods such as coffee beans, peanuts and wheat
- Condiments - many condiments such as soy sauce, tomato sauce, contain very high amounts of salt which can lead to hypertension and the diseases associated with it (including stroke, dementia and cognitive impairment)
- High consumption of foods high in histamine (fermented foods and oxalates (such as beer, chocolate, soy, spinach and nuts), especially in those individuals with histamine tolerance issues.

There are also foods and compounds that have been shown to enhance the health of our brains, improve cognition and reduce brain fog.

42 For more on the effect of gluten on the health of your brain, see "Grain Brain" by Dr David Perlmutter

Enter nootropics.

Nootropics are compounds that enhance brain function. They can be natural or synthetic. They include smart drugs such as Adderall, Ritalin and Modafinil which are sometimes used to treat cognitive disorders such as ADHD and are also used by some individuals with a view to enhancing performance. They cause spikes in certain neurotransmitters such as dopamine, serotonin and norepinephrine and so can lead to imbalances and habit formation.

There are also a growing group of natural compounds that have been shown to protect and enhance brain function that do not carry the risks of synthetic substances.

These include the following:

Caffeine

A time honoured classic 'wake-me-up' and one of my personal favourite nootropics, caffeine stimulates the central nervous system to improve mental alertness. Caffeine is both water and fat soluble and so easily crosses the blood brain barrier. Used in moderation, caffeine can enhance mental performance and protect against Alzheimer's.

Caffeine's structure looks very similar to adenosine which means that it can easily fit into your brain's adenosine receptors, so that you no longer feel the tiredness that is building up. If used in too high doses for too long, your body can create more and more adenosine receptors meaning that you need progressively more and more caffeine to function.

To avoid building up a tolerance, keep caffeine intake moderate or cycle on and off it for days at a time to reset your adenosine receptors. Some people are more sensitive to the effects of caffeine and also process it at different speeds. As mentioned earlier, you can find out your sensitivity by checking your DNA.

L-Theanine

L-Theanine is an amino acid that is found in large quantities in green tea. When taken as a supplement it helps to promote alertness with a sense of calm relaxation at the same time and has often been used by Buddhist monks to enhance meditation.

It also works very well when taken alongside caffeine and using the two together can increase memory, reaction time and reduce mental fatigue.[43]

As mentioned previously, L-Theanine works very well in a 2:1 combination with caffeine, e.g. 200mg of L-Theanine with 100mg of caffeine (one shot of espresso).

CoQ10 & PQQ

As you read earlier, CoQ10 enhances cellular energy production in your mitochondria and PQQ promotes the growth of new mitochondria. The brain's prefrontal cortex contains a high density of mitochondria which is involved in planning, complex cognitive behavior and decision making. Taking supplements containing these can help with smarter, better decision making power!

Bacopa Monnieri

Bacopa is a small water plant native to India and an adaptogen (more on adaptogens in Chapter 5. It has been shown to improve memory in healthy adults. Scientists are unsure of exactly how it

43 https://pubmed.ncbi.nlm.nih.gov/18006208/

works, but it usually takes time to notice the effects. If you are trying bacopa, take it daily for at least 4 weeks to feel the effects.[44]

Alpha GPC

Alpha GPC provides choline which has been shown to increase the production of the neurotransmitter, Acetylcholine. This is needed for learning capacity and boosting memory.

Rhodiola Rosea

Rhodiola Rosea is an ancient flower taken by Vikings before battle. As a powerful adaptogen it has been shown to improve mental and physical stamina, improve resilience to stress and enhance recovery.

Lion's Mane

Lion's Mane, also known as Hericium erinaceus is a type of medicinal mushroom that has powerful antioxidant, anti-inflammatory[45] and immunostimulant properties. It can help to enhance brain health and performance.

Research studies indicate that Lion's Mane may support your brain by stimulating the creation of two important proteins: brain-derived neurotrophic factor (BDNF) and nerve growth factor (NGF) that stimulate the production of new cells and strengthen existing ones.[46]

Nerve cells have a protective sheath around them that helps brain cells communicate with each other. NGF plays an important role in

44 Be aware that bacopa has been shown to suppress sperm production in male mice. https://pubmed.ncbi.nlm.nih.gov/19041444/

45 https://pubmed.ncbi.nlm.nih.gov/26244378/

46 https://pubmed.ncbi.nlm.nih.gov/24266378/, https://link.springer.com/article/10.1023/A:1023963509393, https://www.mdpi.com/1422-0067/19/2/341

forming myelin. BDNF increases neuroplasticity, helping with long term learning and adaptation.

Studies in rodents indicate that Lion's Mane may potentially protect against the effects of Alzheimer's disease[47]. While the exact mechanisms are unclear and lots more research is needed, Lion's Mane may be a useful compound to consider including in your diet if you want to protect your smarts. This is particularly pertinent if, like me you have the APOE4 gene which increases the risk of dementia (more on this below).

Huperzine

Huperzine is derived from Chinese club moss, Huperzia serrata. While the quality of the evidence is low, research suggests that Huperzine may improve neurotransmitter levels and may protect neurons and also improve memory. This also shows potential for treatment for Alzheimer's. Note though that if you are taking medications for Alzheimer's, the Alzheimer's Association recommends that you do not take huperzine.

47 https://pubmed.ncbi.nlm.nih.gov/27350344/, https://www.ncbi.nlm.nih.gov/pmc/articles/PMC5237458/

A NOTE ON LONG TERM BRAIN HEALTH AND DEMENTIA

We are learning more and more about dementia and the way that our brains age. While genetics play a part in risk (as explained below), lifestyle has a big influence.

If you have a double copy of the gene variant APOE2 (one copy from each of your parents), then it would seem that you are one of the lucky people who have a reduced genetic risk of developing Alzheimer's. Most people carry two copies of the gene variant, APOE3 which studies show puts them at around a 9% risk of Alzheimer's.

Like me, 25 percent of Americans (about 75 million people) carry a single copy of APOE4. This puts them at a heightened risk of Alzheimer's disease of about 30% or 3x the risk of individuals who carry two copies of APOE3.

7 million Americans carry 2 copies of APOE4, pushing their risk above 50%.

If you or a family member has or is at greater risk of Alzeimer's disease then I would encourage you to read 'The End of Alzheimer's' by Dr Dale Bredesen. He talks of "36 holes" that are potentially being poked in the "roof" that is our brain.

He groups these into 3 main categories that you should look to optimise if you want to lower your risk of Alzheimer's disease:

1. Prevent and reduce inflammation - avoid inflammatory foods such as processed vegetable oils, processed sugars, insulin resistance, food intolerances and dangerous microbes (from the gut or the mouth).

2. Optimise hormones, trophic factors and nutrients - make sure that you are increasing your 'cognitive reserve' through

BDNF - (with regular exercise and nootropic compounds such as lion's mane, ashwagandha and bacopa monnieri), optimal levels of testosterone and oestradiol, sufficient levels of Vitamin D and folate (found in broccoli and other cruciferous veg).

3. Eliminate toxins - from metals and bio toxins such as mycotoxins from mould. They can encourage the build up of amyloid plaque which Dr Dale Bredesen explains may be produced to protect neutrons from toxic damage. Avoid toxic exposure, prioritising detoxification through consumption of cruciferous vegetables, ensure adequate hydration, take a regular sauna and make sure you are producing enough glutathione.

Another area to focus on that I now ruthlessly prioritise since discovering I have a copy of APOE4 - is sleep. Revisit Chapter 2 on sleep if you want to refresh your memory on how to enhance your sleep.

RETHINK > > >

TRADITIONAL THINKING:

- The calories in, calories out equation determines our weight.
- As we get older, we naturally gain weight, in particular, abdominal weight gain.
- Our genes dictate our destiny.
- Aging is a natural process over which we have no control.

RETHINK:

- Food is medicine. It is information that communicates to our cells and affects the expression of our genes (epigenetics) in real time.
- We can personalise our diet to our genes and take active steps to optimise their expression to live a healthier, longer life.
- By eating an abundance of wild and organic plants, superfoods, healthy fats and moderate protein with targeted supplementation we can increase our energy, health, longevity and create a high performance brain and body.

In a sense, we can live younger for longer.

Chapter 5
STRESS, RESILIENCE AND RE-COVERY

"The time to relax is when you don't have time for it"
Sydney J. Harris

If you want to live younger for longer, one thing is clear; you need to manage stress. As you learnt in the previous chapter, wild plants become stronger and more resilient because of stress. As humans we need stress to grow stronger and become more resilient. Stress can be a force for both good and bad.

What is stress?

It can be divided into two main types:

- **Physical stress** - such as the stress you get from working out or training hard
- **Mental stress** - that which arises when you are required to perform, such as to give a speech or tackle financial or other concerns.

Mental stress has long been talked about as damaging to health and performance, but new research shows this not to be the case. It can in fact be performance enhancing.

Kelly McGonigal, author of ***'The Upside of Stress'*** provides a useful definition of stress:

"Stress is what happens when something that you care about is at stake".

She explains that "stress and meaning are inextricably linked. You don't stress about things you don't care about, and you can't create a meaningful life without experiencing some stress".

It is the things and people that we care most about that we are most likely to feel stressed about. As such, if we are to live a meaningful life we must accept stress as an integral part of it. The question then arises; when is stress good for you and when does stress become too much?

To understand this we need to first look at the Threat Response. You may have heard of this described as the fight-or-flight response. As Emily Fletcher, author of 'Stress Less, Accomplish More' (and guest on my podcast, High Performance Health) explains "stress makes you stupid"; or at least it's the threat response that makes you stupid.

When we are faced with something that engages our threat response, a number of physiological things happen, including the following:

- the digestive system floods with acid
- our blood thickens and coagulates
- our vision reduces
- our bowels may evacuate
- our adrenal levels increase
- cortisol levels increase
- our Immune system is deprioritised by the body and moved to the back burner.

The immune system and the adrenal system do not function well at the same time. If you imagine a situation where you are faced with the threat of a sabre toothed tiger and a virus at the same time, your body needs to prioritise fighting or fleeing from the sabre toothed tiger first, rather than responding to the virus.

When the threat response is engaged we lose the thinking power of our prefrontal cortex, with the amygdala (a collection of cells at the base of the brain involved in emotion and fear) firing and taking control.

It is easy to assume that individuals who seem to be in control of stress and who even perform at their highest level in stressful situations are somehow calmer. Think of elite level athletes such as tennis player, Roger Federer or golfer, Tiger Woods. It's easy to assume that these individuals are much calmer under pressure when in reality this has been shown not to be the case. What they are doing is engaging with the stressful situation in a very different way. Instead of engaging the ***Threat Response*** they are engaging the ***Challenge Response*** and this is driven by their perception of stress. When you engage the Challenge Response you are still experiencing stress. As Kelly McGonigal explains, just like the fight-or-flight response "your heart rate still rises, your adrenaline spikes, your muscles and brain get more fuel and the feel good chemicals surge. But it differs from a fight-or-flight response in a few important ways: You feel focused, but not fearful. You also release a different ratio of stress hormones, including high levels of DHEA which helps you recover and learn from stress". The challenge response gives you energy to meet the demands being placed upon you and helps you to perform under pressure.

As Tiger Woods is reported as saying; "The day I'm not nervous is the day I quit...That's the greatest thing about it - just to feel that rush."

To initiate the Challenge Response instead of the Threat Response, you need to change your mindset around stress. Many people believe that stress is harmful and that it depletes their health and vitality. High performers often perceive stress differently - they believe that stress is enhancing and they use it to improve their performance and productivity, to improve their health and vitality and to facilitate learning and growth.

How do they do this? They change their perception of, and attitude towards stress.

Here is an example of how to reframe stress and move from the the threat response to the challenge response:

RESPONSE	THOUGHT	ACTION	RESULT	EFFECT
Challenge	"I'm excited to use this (to make an impact) and I have the resources I need to deal with it"	Engage with it	Increased Performance	Easier to connect with others, better health outcomes.
Threat	"I'm anxious or nervous that I won't be able to cope"	Avoid it	Decreased Performance	Associated with heightened inflammation and blood pressure, harder to connect with others

Acknowledge you care about it and step into it

The perception of stress is extremely important. Many people who feel stressed believe that they should try to calm themselves down. Most people are familiar with the stress that they feel before speaking publicly in front of a large group of people. The instinct is often to try to calm down, but science shows that another approach may be preferable. Harvard Business School professor Alison Wood Brooks decided to test which response was optimal. She brought people into a laboratory and asked them to prepare for giving a speech. Immediately before the speech half of the participants were told to say to themselves "I am calm" and the other half to say "I am excited" while embracing the anxiety. Both groups of people felt nervous but the group that told themselves they were excited and embraced their anxiety reported feeling more confident and better able to handle the pressure. This played out in their performance as they gave better speeches.

The people who were watching the speeches rated the group of excited speakers' as more confident, persuasive and competent than the participants who had tried to calm down. McGonigal explains that welcoming stress can boost confidence and improve performance.

It can seem difficult and counterintuitive to embrace stress in this way; this is where knowing the importance of your values comes into play. It is in understanding your values that allows you to truly know what you care about in life.

One of the most important things you can do to manage stress and improve your health is to journal about your values. In a study carried out in the 1990s upon a group of Stanford students, they were asked to keep journals about their most important values and how their day-to-day activities related to those values. Another group was asked to write about the good things that happened to them. The students that wrote about their values were in better health and better spirits at the end of the three-week experiment. After analysing more than 2,000 pages from the students' journals the researchers came to the conclusion that writing about values helps students to see meaning in their lives. By writing about their values the students no longer saw the stressful experience of their writing assignments as hassles to endure. Instead, the assignments became an expression of the students' values.

What can we take away from this? That stress is part of a meaningful life and that cultivating a mindset of meaning is protective of our health and performance enhancing.

> In order to better understand our values, purpose and meaning, Kelly McGonigal asks us to journal regularly, reflecting upon four questions:
>
> - What kind of positive impact do you want to have on the people around you?
> - What mission in life or at work most inspires you?
> - What do you want to contribute to the world?

- What change do you want to create?

From this we can see that the mindset we have around stress is extremely powerful as an influence upon both our health and our performance. This is also explored in Ian Robertson's book, 'The Stress Test'. Robertson talks about how stress can make you not just stronger, but better. It can boost your performance so long as you do not worry about or doubt your ability. When that's the response then it has the opposite effect and actually weakens your performance.

Stress is not always bad. If used correctly in the right dose, stress is a peak performance elixir.

People often talk about stress as something outside of themselves, labelling things like school or work as stressful. The issue with this approach is that it takes away your control. If on the other hand, you reclaim stress as something that is happening within you, it immediately opens doors for ways for you to change the way that you think about stress and respond to it. It enables you to use the stress as a catalyst to change - to take positive actions for learning, growth and connecting with others.

Studies show that if you believe that your stress is harmful, it is more likely to be harmful. If stress is harmful, believing that it is harmful seems to amplify the damaging consequences of the stress.

If you accept, embrace and welcome stress in ways that demonstrate that you value it then it changes you and empowers you to support your goals. This is why knowing your values and being clear on them is so important.

Does this mean that you can put yourself in stressful situations on a constant basis and expect to have optimised health and high performance? This is unlikely, as you need to factor in recovery as a necessary part of the puzzle. Recovery is one of the most underrated but important areas of health and performance.

Stress can be good in its many forms; it can make us physically and mentally stronger and it can help us to perform better. But if we want sustained higher performance we need to include significant periods of recovery in our lives too.

RECOVERY

One of the most overlooked and underrated areas of health optimization and peak performance is recovery, certainly in the world of business and corporations. Athletes however, approach this in a completely different way.

I often coach my clients on the importance of treating yourself like an athlete to optimise your health for sustained high performance. Stress is an essential part of high performance, it is necessary for survival and it can be used as a catalyst for growth. Stress can also be the ultimate peak performance elixir.

Athletes use stress in a positive way to get bigger, stronger or faster. But any elite coach will confirm that an athlete doesn't get stronger in the gym, they get stronger from the adaptations that take place during rest and recovery. In the same way that athletes train hard, they recover harder. If we as individuals want to perform at our best in our vocation, our family life and our hobbies then we need to match sessions of intense activity with periods of intense recovery.

As we get older, those times of recovery become ever more important. We may have once pushed ourselves in our twenties and early thirties through repeated periods of energetic growth and work, dedicated to being a success. As we move through our late thirties, forties, fifties and beyond it is simply not possible to sustain the same high level of performance without taking a break regularly.

We have competing demands and particularly in our forties, many of us are combining a busy career with raising children. There is no longer the opportunity to go at things hard and then recover lying on a beach for two weeks as we may have done in our twenties.

Stress is fundamental to growth, but in driving that growth and enhancing performance we can learn a lot from sports science.

There are three common concepts within sports science:

- Functional overreaching (FOR)
- Non-functional overreaching (NFOR)
- Overtraining syndrome (OTS).

The right way to encourage growth is to use functional overreaching (FOR). FOR is when you experience a short term drop in performance at the end of a training block. This applies to protocols in strength training, aerobic training or any team sport. It also applies when you have completed a significant project or period of intense work. While you may have overreached yourself, if done functionally with sufficient recovery, you will have enabled your personal growth and development. It does not have significant long term adverse effects on your immune system, your health or your mood.

When you push too far, fatigue and exhaustion can set in and this can weaken your performance. This is when you experience lowered energy levels and a drop in motivation. This type of overreaching, known in the athletic world as non functional overreaching (NFOR) is when you have pushed too far and/or you haven't engaged in sufficient recovery.

NFOR happens when you don't build in sufficient periods of recovery on a quarterly, monthly, weekly and even intra-daily basis. I'll explain more on how to build in effective recovery in a moment.

For now, understand that if you dip into your equivalent of NFOR it can take weeks to regain your prior high performance levels. To use the analogy of an athlete, this is akin to going 'all out' in every workout. It eventually leads to stagnation and symptoms of fatigue.

If you ignore the signs and push on for long enough, powering yourself with caffeine and other stimulants without taking the time to properly recover, you risk moving into a third stage known as overtraining syndrome (OTS).

This is where you are either working too hard or not recovering enough (or both), on a sustained basis. It can lead to biological, hormonal and neurochemical impairments. Essentially you end up with a weaker body and brain as a result. The difficulty with overtraining syndrome (or in the corporate equivalent - 'burnout' or as it is more scientifically termed, HPA Axis Dysfunction) is that in my experience, it can be very difficult to turn that ship around. Many people who've experienced chronic fatigue syndrome will be familiar with how difficult it can be to overcome this and how the smallest stimulus can trigger the onset of symptoms even after you feel you've made a recovery.

From my own experience with burnout and clinical depression, I know how difficult it is to turn the 'burnout tanker' around, and so I make a constant effort to ensure that I am getting sufficient recovery.

This enables me to achieve far higher levels of productivity and success than I would if I simply pushed on regardless. It also means that by recovering on a consistent basis I don't have the need to take long periods out.

"Energy, not time, is the fundamental currency of high performance"
- Jim Loehr and Tony Schwartz.

In their book, ***'The Power of Full Engagement'***, Jim Loehr and Tony Schwartz talk about the four principles of full engagement. These are as follows:

- **Principle 1:** Full engagement requires us to draw on four separate but related sources of energy: physical, emotional, mental and spiritual.

- **Principle 2:** Energy diminishes with both overuse and underuse and so we must balance energy expenditure with intermittent energy renewal.
- **Principle 3:** To build capacity we must push beyond our normal limits in the same way that elite athletes do.
- **Principle 4:** We need positive energy rituals - highly specific routines that we use for managing energy.

We need to make sure that we are pushing hard enough such that we are functionally overreaching and stressing ourselves in a positive way that facilitates positive adaptations in our health and our performance. To do this we need to work hard and recover hard. Most people neither push themselves hard enough or spend enough time in recovery.

If you have managed so far to follow all of the steps in this book in optimising your sleep, nutrition and movement you will be a long way towards optimising your four sources of energy - your physical, emotional, mental and spiritual health. To become fully optimised you need to build in energy enhancing rituals that facilitate recovery and relaxation.

To manage our energy effectively we need first to understand the rhythms of life. These are the biological rhythms of the natural cycle of change within our bodily functions and chemicals. There are four biological rhythms:

- **Circadian rhythm:** the 24-hour cycle that includes physiological and behavioral rhythms like sleeping and waking
- **Diurnal rhythm:** the circadian rhythm that is synced with day and night
- **Infradian rhythms:** biological rhythms that last longer than 24 hours such as a menstrual cycle
- **Ultradian rhythms:** biological rhythms that have a shorter period and a higher frequency than circadian rhythm.

I looked at the importance of aligning with our circadian rhythm in Chapter 2 (on sleep). In Chapter 3 (on movement) I talked about adapting nutrition and exercise protocols according to the female menstrual cycle. The other rhythm that is important here is your ultradian rhythm. First discovered by Nathan Kleitman, a groundbreaking sleep researcher, the ultradian rhythm is the 90 minute cycle which you progress through in the five stages of sleep (see Chapter 2). It has also been found that we have this 90-minute pattern in our days, and that we move from higher to lower alertness during this time. Research carried out upon top performers indicates that they work in alignment with this 90-minute rhythm, generally working or training in 90 minute blocks with 20-minute recoveries in between.

In a widely cited study of prodigious violinists, psychologist Anders Ericsson found that the top performers all had the same characteristics in their practice. They each practised in the morning for 3 sessions and each session was 90 minutes or less. They also had a break between each session. The study showed that the top performers engaged in highly deliberate and focused practice and that very few were able to engage in practice for more than 4 or 5 hours at a time.

The pattern among top performers seems to be focus > rest > focus > rest. It demonstrates that by observing the ebb and flow of concentration and focus you can actually achieve more.

The way to do this is to build in specific recovery periods during the course of your day. In Chapter 2 we discussed your genetic chronotype and how it can determine whether you are an early morning or evening person. Understanding this can help you to schedule your most productive and creative work at the right time of day.

As a morning person, I find that the most productive hours for focusing upon demanding tasks is between 8.00am and 2pm. It is for this reason that I block out my diary in the morning and focus on my key performance tasks such as writing and producing content, leaving less cognitively demanding tasks for the afternoon. I work in 90 minute blocks of extreme productivity between 8:00am and 2pm with regular breaks every 30 minutes or so to get up, change position, stretch, do some jumping jacks or skipping.

In the afternoon, I will do more social tasks such as podcast interviews, Facebook lives or admin work.

To do your best work you need to get into a 'flow state'. Steven Koetler explains in his book 'The Rise of Superhuman' that attention is most engaged when there is a specific relationship between the difficulty of a task and the ability to perform that task. He explains that flow is near the emotional midpoint between boredom and anxiety - the point where the "task is hard enough to make us stretch but not hard enough to make us snap". He explains that this is about 4% greater than your current skill set.

How to Know if You're Pushing Too Hard

One of the best ways to track how hard you're pushing is to look at a measurement known as Heart Rate Variability (HRV).

HRV is the physiological variation in time interval between successive heartbeats in milliseconds. A normal, healthy heart doesn't beat evenly like a metronome. There is constant variation which we are not usually aware of. Generally speaking, the longest intervals take place when you exhale, and the shortest intervals when you inhale. It is different to your heart rate which is the number of beats per minute. The variation between beats (HRV) is influenced by a number of factors including underlying health status, exercise, hormones, gender, metabolic processes, neurological processes, stress and recovery.

To understand HRV we first need to understand our nervous system and heart rate.

We have two main branches to our nervous system: the Central Nervous System (CNS) and the Peripheral Nervous System (PNS). The PNS is divided into three separate subsystems; the somatic, autonomic and enteric nervous systems. When looking at heart rate variability we are concerned with the part of our nervous system that regulates very important systems in our body, including the heart, our respiration rate and digestion.

The autonomic nervous system has two main branches - the parasympathetic (rest) and sympathetic (activation) branches. Higher heart rate variability is an indicator that both branches are functioning; in particular this applies to the parasympathetic nervous system. When the rest-related parasympathetic branch is active and the sympathetic branch is inactive, your heart rate is generally lower and your HRV is higher. The sympathetic and parasympathetic nervous system cannot operate at the same time. When you are stressed this can lead to a disengagement of parasympathetic activity with much greater activation of the sympathetic branch. This leads to elevated heart rate and lowered HRV.

High HRV means that your body is responsive to both sets of inputs (parasympathetic and sympathetic). This is a good sign that your nervous system is balanced and that your body is able to adapt to its changing environment and perform at its best.

On the other hand, if you have low HRV then one branch is dominating. This is usually (but not always) the sympathetic nervous system and it is sending stronger signals to your heart than the other.

This is a good thing when you want your body to be in a sympathetic state and respond to a more intense situation - for example, when you are giving a presentation or running a race. However, when you are not doing something active, low HRV indicates that your body is working hard for some other reason. You may be fighting off an infection, maybe you're dehydrated, overstressed or tired.

When this happens you have fewer resources available to dedicate towards more stimulating activities such as exercising or giving a presentation at work.

Measuring your heart rate variability at night or upon waking is a good way of assessing how parasympathetically engaged you are.

What Can You Learn From Your HRV?

Heart rate variability is one of the indicators of the state of your health, fitness, recovery and readiness. I measure my HRV each night with my Oura Ring which combines the data to give me a 'readiness score' in the morning. While this is only one metric of many that I track, I find it very useful as it gives me an indication of when I am pushing too hard.

HRV is Highly Individualized

HRV is an extremely sensitive metric. It fluctuates greatly throughout the day, week and month. It also fluctuates greatly from one person to the next. Many people that track their HRV often wonder "What should my HRV be?" and "How does my HRV compare to others?"

Generally speaking, younger people have higher HRV than older people and men often have slightly higher HRV than women. Elite athletes usually have higher HRV than the average person, particularly endurance athletes who tend to have higher HRV than strength-based athletes.

However, there is no absolute rule over what is good or bad. There are lots of extremely fit and healthy individuals who have an HRV that is regularly in the forties. What's important is the ability to modulate your own HRV.

The best way to understand your HRV, is to check it regularly and notice trends. The question you want to be asking yourself is "What is a good HRV for me?" and "How can I enhance my HRV?".

It's worth pointing out that HRV values, like your overall health and fitness are multifactorial, so you should be paying attention to other things such as how you feel on the whole, your nutrition, your sleep, your movement and so-on. HRV is a good indicator, but it's still just one indicator. You should not rely too heavily on HRV or any one single measurement alone.

If you are tracking HRV there are a few things to pay attention to:

1. Find your HRV Baseline: That is to say, your typical HRV when you're feeling as you generally feel on an average day. Your baseline is the starting point for your HRV explorations.

2. After you have established your baseline you can start to monitor how your health, nutrition, movement, stress levels and lifestyle are affecting your HRV.

If you notice your HRV going down this may mean that something is burdening your body or your mind. You may be overtraining or you may be going through a particularly stressful time. If your body or mind is under stress it may be too much to add to it, even with good forms of stress (known as hormesis - the adaptive response of biological systems to moderate stress). You can read more on this later.

Think of your capacity to take on stress like a glass. If you start half full, you will be able to take on less additional stress before you are overloaded. If on the other hand, you are practising good recovery techniques such as breathwork and meditation, your baseline stress may be very low which enables you to add in moderate stressors such as high intensity or endurance exercise or cold thermogenesis such as a cold swim or plunge.

If your HRV goes up, it suggests that you are under less stress or perhaps you are engaging in practices that are good for your body and/or mind.

Factors that can affect your HRV scores include the following:

Biological Factors	Lifestyle / Environmental Factors
Age	Hydration
Gender	Nutrition
Genetics	Sleep
Immune System	Circadian Rhythm
Chronic Health Conditions	Alcohol
Breathing Rate	Volume & Intensity of Training
Hormones	Stress levels
	Recovery / Rest
	Level of Demands

WAYS TO IMPROVE HRV AND ENHANCE RECOVERY

There are a number of ways to improve your HRV and enhance the functioning of your parasympathetic nervous system. These methods are all good for helping to optimise your health further and live younger for longer.

EXERCISE

Exercise has been shown to improve HRV but the dose and type of exercise is important as is taking account of your current HRV levels. Studies in recreational endurance athletes show that those with low HRV may respond more positively to a higher volume of low intensity training rather than high intensity workouts such as interval training. Those with higher HRV may respond more positively to higher intensity training.

If you notice that your HRV is lower than normal or is on a downward trajectory, it suggests that your sympathetic nervous system may be overstimulated. This could be as a result of too much exercise or it could be down to too much load overall. If you are going through a particularly stressful time at work or you have just welcomed a new baby into your family and you are still trying to continue to train at previous levels, you may be putting too much strain on your body. Focusing on lower intensity exercise such as Low Intensity Steady State (LISS) exercise, or yoga may help to recover HRV levels. Training in zones 1 and 2 of Maximum Heart Rate (MHR) are effective ways of improving HRV and lowering resting pulse.

When your HRV is low it is a good opportunity to engage in recovery practices such as flexibility and mobility work. As your

HRV starts to recover you can go back to pushing yourself again, while carefully monitoring your readiness. The key thing is to train intelligently and give your body the recovery it needs. Most people benefit from one day of recovery each week, while individuals over the age of 45 often require at least two.

RESTORATIVE PRACTICES

Restorative practices that engage the parasympathetic nervous system such as mediation and breathwork can help you recover and improve HRV. Pranayama (for example) is a form of rhythmic breathing that has been shown to enhance the parasympathetic nervous system.

More detail is provided on these below.

SLEEP

Adequate sleep is very important for enhancing HRV. In particular you should make sure that you go to bed early enough and practice good sleep hygiene so that you are getting enough deep or slow wave sleep. This is the time when growth hormone and testosterone is released which is important for healthy HRV. For more information on how to optimise your sleep, refer back to Chapter 2.

COLD SHOWERS (AND OTHER COLD THERMOGENESIS)

Cold exposure has been shown to improve HRV. Great ways to engage in cold exposure include taking a swim in a local lake or river, visiting a cryotherapy chamber, or taking an ice bath or a cold shower. To start getting the benefits of cold exposure, start by turning the tap to fully cold for 15 to 30 seconds at the end of your usual shower.

EAT AN ANTI-INFLAMMATORY DIET

Pro-inflammatory foods increase inflammation and can affect HRV levels. If you are trying to improve HRV, limit your intake of alcohol, processed foods, foods that are high in omega-6 fatty acids (such as roasted seeds and nuts) and focus on eating colourful foods high in antioxidants (such as cherries, berries, broccoli). You should also eat larger quantities of omega-3 rich foods (such as oily fish, walnuts and flaxseeds) which are anti-inflammatory. Finally, consider taking natural herbal anti-inflammatories (such as turmeric, garlic and ginger) or take a curcumin and/or omega-3 supplement.

ADAPTOGENIC HERBS

If your HRV levels are falling, or you are experiencing a high level of stress, it may be time to start taking some adaptogenic herbal blends. Adaptogens have stimulant properties that help to counter the effects of stress. Examples of adaptogenic herbs are:

- **Ashwagandha** - a herb used in ayurvedic medicine that has been used for over 3000 years to relieve stress, increase energy levels and improve concentration.
- **Ginseng** - a tonic that is used to support stress and energy, and has been shown to enhance heart rate variability.
- **Borage** - the herb, rather than the oil, which has been used to strengthen and restore the adrenal cortex.
- **Eleutherococcus senticosus** - similar to ginseng in adaptogenic activity. It is also used to support stress and energy.

- **Liquorice** - has also been shown to support adrenal function and is thought to revitalise the adrenal glands.
- **Gotu kola** - a member of the parsley family and regarded in India as possibly one of the most spiritual of all of the herbs. It is used by the Yogiz to improve meditation and is said to develop the Crown chakra which is the energy centre at the top of the head. It is also said to balance the right and left hemispheres of the brain. In Ayurvedic medicine it is also regarded as one of the most rejuvenative herbs alongside bacopa monnieri.
- **Bacopa monnieri** - another adaptogenic herb. Research suggests that it may help to reduce stress and anxiety by reducing cortisol levels and elevating your mood.

Adaptogenic herbs can also affect hormone levels and so to personalise your approach for best results, work with a qualified practitioner.

Each of the recovery techniques in this chapter should help to improve heart rate variability and engage the relaxation response. As Herbert Benson writes in his book ***'The Relaxation Revolution'*** there isn't a single correct approach for triggering the relaxation response. The most important thing is the mind-body response that's induced. Benson explains that there are three key things that you should focus on daily:

1. To break the pattern of everyday thoughts
2. To assume a passive attitude or an 'ah-well' attitude towards distracting thoughts
3. To devote 12 to 15 minutes towards triggering your relaxation response.

The way in which you trigger the relaxation response is less relevant than the practice itself. It doesn't really matter whether you use a mantra meditation, breath work, yoga or prayer. Benson explains that all techniques yield the same gene expression, namely the changes in gene activity that are the opposite of those associated with stress.

MEDITATION

In Chapter 4 you learned about how you can use nutrition to influence the expression of your genes. Meditation is another way you can become an epigenetic engineer. Epigenetics literally means 'above the genes'. It is the impact of your environment on your genes. In his book 'You are the Placebo', Dr Joe Dispenza explains:

"With every thought you think, every emotion you feel and every event you experience, you're acting as an epigenetic engineer of your own cells. You control your destiny".

In the book, Dispenza dives deep into the research of epigenetics and explains that soliciting the relaxation response produces changes in gene expression after just one meditation. This is the case both among people who are new to meditation and experienced practitioners alike.

There have been over 6,000 peer-reviewed scientific studies on meditation. Jonathan Haidt, author of 'The Happiness Hypothesis' describes meditation as a "magic pill" for reducing anxiety and contentment.

After struggling with clinical depression for over 10 years, there are a number of practices that helped me on my journey to recovery. If I could name a single practice above all others that has helped me improve my mood, lower anxiety and help me stay emotionally balanced, it's meditation.

Meditation is a game changer. Let me say that again - **meditation is a game changer**. And that's coming from someone who can't sit still and has to grapple constantly with the monkey that is my mind.

Meditation is a performance enhancer. It's one of the most powerful practices for getting in touch with your inner self and for finding the bridge between your inner world and the outer world that you want to create. It's an entry point into your future reality. It's the place from which you can create and make your wildest dreams come true. It's the stairway to manifesting your ideal life.

It's also a wonderful way to stimulate your parasympathetic nervous system and engage in a period of recovery. While some of the most powerful times to meditate are when you first wake up and when you go to bed (more on this below), meditation can also be used as a post-lunch rejuvenator to power afternoon productivity.

Think of your brain as a computer. As you think different thoughts or do different things, it's as though you are opening new windows on your browser on your computer. After an hour or two, your computer is slower and less responsive. So much of that computing power is being used to run those open windows. This is essentially what is happening to our brain.

Emily Fletcher, author of ***'Stress Less, Accomplish More'*** explains that by the time we are 20 years old we have approximately 10 million Precognitive Commitments (PCCs) which are like open windows on our 'brain computer". Emily explains that every time you've been a little bit stressed or entered into a little bit of a fight or flight state, it's as though you've left a little open window on your brain computer. All of those open windows are keeping you from being as productive as you could be, and from performing at the top of your game. She explains that meditation allows you to close down those windows, but before you can do that you need to maximize them. When they are operating in the background she describes it as if they are all draining you of energy.

She explains that many of the world's top performers including professional athletes, world class hedge fund managers such as

Ray Dalio and even Oprah Winfrey, are all meditators. They do this, not because they have endless amounts of time to spare but because it actually gives them time back in their day and enhanced performance.

Meditation is like hitting a reset button for your brain. People often worry about whether they are any good at meditation or whether they've had a good or a bad meditation but I love the way Emily Fletcher explains that the purpose of meditation is so that "you can get really good at life". No one cares whether you are a good meditator or not. It's about how you perform when you come out of that meditation that makes a difference and that's why top performers use meditation as a brain reset button. Meditation works very well as an intra-day method of recovery. Her meditation technique, Ziva meditation, can be used twice a day to help you perform at the top of your game.

You can try this after lunch and witness for yourself the improved productivity and concentration that you will enjoy in the afternoon. I found a great time to perform this meditation is at around 2pm when you're starting to experience that post-lunch dip in energy.

One of the things that I love about meditation is that it's so simple and unjudging. This is one of the most important parts of any meditation practice - that you should not be judging your thoughts. Emily uses the analogy of a bouncer, explaining that your job is not to be the bouncer at the party. Your job is not to decide which thoughts should or shouldn't be present. During meditation your job is simply to acknowledge the thoughts as they come into your head and return to your mantra or guided practice, letting each thought glide in and out. If instead you focus or attach on any one thought then you have moved from meditation into contemplation.

That's not to say that you can expect your mind to be quiet. In fact, the purpose of meditation doesn't have to be to quieten the mind. The mind by its very nature wants to think and be busy.

Emily Fletcher explains that "thinking during meditation is actually an indicator that some stress is leaving the body", explaining that this is where the healing happens. When those thoughts bubble up, it is stress exiting your nervous system". The most important thing to remember, Emily explains, is that "a deep meditation is no better for you than a shallow meditation."

I love this, as it removes any sense of competition that you may have with yourself regarding whether you are or aren't a good meditator. She explains that a deep meditation means that the body is getting deep rest and a shallow meditation means the body is releasing stress in the form of thought. One is not better for you than the other. The purpose of meditation is to "de-excite our nervous system".

As someone who has been meditating for the last few years, I notice that my ability to bring calm focused presence to what I am doing outside of meditation has greatly improved.

FORMS OF MEDITATION

There are many different forms of meditation including vedic, vipassana, yogic, spiritual and transcendental.

Transcendental Meditation (TM), is a type of meditation that is taught one on one. In practising this form of meditation you focus on a mantra. It is said to be the most effective techniques for 'transcending', which means 'going beyond the normal or physical level', connecting you to the dynamic power of nature's silent, restful alertness. There have been thousands of studies done on TM and its ability to deliver a potentially greater range of mental, physical and spiritual benefits. Meta-analyses (statistical analysis of multiple research studies) have found that TM is very effective in producing a range of results, including reducing anxiety, lowering blood pressure, reducing addiction and increasing self-actualisation.

TM involves neither concentration nor training the mind. Innocence is said to be key in this form of practice, for the reason that as evaluation, control or manipulation can leave you caught up in thinking and prevent the act of transcendence.

In TM, alpha brain waves (characteristic of reduced mental activity and relaxation) permeate the whole brain, which receives more oxygen as a result. Blood flow to the front of the brain (which is coordinating activity) is increased while the core of the brain is quieter, indicating alertness in the midst of deep rest. This is indicative of getting into the state of transcendental or pure consciousness.

Transcendental Meditation is designed to be done twice a day for 20 minutes. It is individualised and taught one-to-one. If you are looking for online guided meditations that can help you learn to reach a 'transcendental state' there are some great courses, apps and online programmes available.

Once you learn a meditation technique you can use it anywhere, at any time. One of the powerful results of a consistent meditation practice is that it provides an entry point to the subconscious mind and the ability to change unwanted programmes you are running unconsciously.

The brain operates in a range of different brain wave states. When the conscious mind is operating functionally during the course of the day it is in a beta state. When someone is anxious they move into a fight or flight mode and their brain waves move into high beta. High beta is a highly aroused, active state. This is when the HPA Axis kicks in and signals the release of cortisol and adrenaline. These hormones constrict blood flow in the prefrontal cortex where our logic and reasoning centres are located. Blood flow is redirected to our older, reflexive, reptilian brain where instinctive action originates. When you quieten the HPA Axis, you are in a position to rewire your brain and create 'a new self'. This is not just a great way to relieve stress and calm you down but also a superpower as an entry point to achieving your wildest goals.

How can you open the door to your subconscious? Dr Joe Dispenza says "we get there on a brain wave". Specifically, we need to drop down from beta brain waves into the slower, more mellow brain wave states of alpha and theta.Theta, Dr Dispenza tells us, is the "key to your own subconscious kingdom".

Scientists can measure brain waves using an electroencephalogram (EEG). An EEG measures your brain waves in cycles per second (CPS). The table below shows the CPS range of different brain wave states:

Brain Wave Type	CPS	Characteristics
Delta	½-4	Deep, unconscious sleep
Theta	5-7	Deep, comfortable sleep
Alpha	8-13	Meditation REM Sleep
Beta	14-40	Conscious, aware state

Jose Silva, author of 'The Silva Mind Control Method of Mental Dynamics' explains that the more agitated we are, the higher our brain waves' CPS. When our CPS goes above 21 we are in a state of agitation, stress or inability to focus. When our brain waves are above 21 cycles per second we effectively cut off all creative thinking. If we can bring it down to 19 we can enter the mythical land of genius! This is where we are our most creative.

Meditation is one way to slow our brain waves from beta to alpha. In his guided meditations Dr Dispenza teaches listeners to do this by sensing the vastness of the space around them to "become no body, no one, no thing, no where, in no time". As consciousness, rather than your body, you are no longer picking up the sensory information around you and so you are no longer living by the hormones of stress. In that state, you are neither asleep nor awake. Instead you are able to reach transcendence.

When we go to sleep at night, the release of melatonin helps us to move from beta to alpha to theta and to delta brain waves. When we wake up in the morning, the reverse happens via the release of serotonin.

And so, morning and evening - when you first wake up and before you go to bed - may be two of the best times to practice meditation. These are the times of day when the door to the subconscious mind naturally opens up.

The Silva method uses a simple breathing technique to slow down and get into an alpha brain wave state quickly and easily. This is accessed through the breath.

To do this you need to find a comfortable sitting position with your spine straight. Next close your eyes and take a deep breath in. Exhale. Inhale again and then on the exhale say silently in your mind "three, three, three". Take another deep breath in and then exhale slowly saying "two, two, two". Finally take one last deep breath in and on the exhale say "one, one, one".

If you're particularly agitated then you can start this process at 10 and count down. You should focus on nice deep long breaths and you will slow down your thoughts as you move your brain waves from beta to alpha. In common with Emily Fletcher's Ziva meditation technique, this is both a relaxation and a performance tool that you can use anywhere and at any time.

It is particularly helpful when you are feeling anxious or agitated. In their book, 'The Silva Mind Control Method Of Mental Dynamics', Jose Silva and Burt Goldman explain that "the only way to get stress out of your being is to let in relaxation" just as "there is no way to get dark out of a room other than to let light in". Silva and Goldman elaborate that stress is not caused by problems but by one's attitude towards the problem. They offer one of the simplest and easiest overviews of how to be happy, condensing it into 5 rules:

1. If you like something, enjoy it.
2. If you don't like something, avoid it.
3. If you don't like something and can't avoid it, change it.
4. If you can't or choose not to to avoid or change something you don't like, then accept it.
5. You accept something by changing your perception of it.

How can you put this into practice? Silva and Godman give a great example of a student that attended one of their seminars.

On leaving for a lunch break the student discovered that someone had smashed into the bumper of his car. Instead of complaining about what happened all through lunch, the student practiced acceptance. He realised that he didn't like the fact that his bumper had been smashed but he could neither change nor avoid it, and so he accepted what it would cost (he figured out it would cost around $250 to fix his bumper). He changed his perception by celebrating the fact that in smashing his car, the person had given him the opportunity to set a fun financial goal for himself. The student decided to set a goal of earning 3 times the amount of the cost to fix his bumper.

Happiness is always a choice and it is up to us to create the most empowering story that we can out of the events that happen to us. This brings me on to another powerful practice that enables stress reduction - that is the power of gratitude.

Gratitude

Gratitude is a way of appreciating what you have, instead of always reaching for something new in the hope of it making you happier or believing that you can't be happy until every physical and material need is met. Gratitude helps people to focus on what they have instead of what they don't have.

When you introduce a daily practice of conscious, mindful gratitude you will notice the positivity flow into your life, along with a greater amount of empathy and altruism.

In positive psychology research, gratitude is strongly and consistently associated with greater levels of happiness and health. It helps people feel more positive emotions, enjoy good experiences, enhance their health, deal with adversity and build strong relationships both at work and at home.

Research also shows that grateful people experience less aches and pains and are more likely to take care of their health, exercise regularly and live longer. A gratitude practice has also been shown to strengthen immunity and help you sleep better too.

Practising gratitude was an instrumental part of me overcoming clinical depression and learning to reframe events as 'happening for me', rather than 'happening to me'. Although practising gratitude can feel contrived at first, it's a mental state that gets stronger with use and practice. There are many ways to practice gratitude and one of my favourite ways in our household is to name one to three things that we are grateful for at our family dinner in the evening. This is the time when the five of us come together to talk about our day and focus on what we are grateful for. It is an experience that we really cherish. It is also a very calming practice and a great way to bookend your day.

Another way to do this is with a gratitude journal. I like the Five Minute Journal which involves a morning and evening practice where you list three things that you are grateful for in the morning and then at the end of the day, note down three things that went well and something that could have made the day even better. This helps to set the tone for the day ahead, celebrates what you have achieved at the end of that day as well as encouraging a positive outlook for the following one.

BREATHWORK

Your breath is one area that you can choose to consciously control and leave to the unconscious control of the autonomic nervous system. It is an entry point to the parasympathetic nervous system and using your breath is one of the fastest ways to quell anxiety and enter a more parasympathetic state.

There are a number of different ways to do this, but here are a few of my favorite techniques that you can try integrating into your day to enhance relaxation and minimise stress.

Buteyko Breathing

Buteyko breathing was created by a Russian physician of the same name. Buteyko breathing helps you correct ratios of oxygen to carbon dioxide in the blood. Many people over breathe in oxygen and over exhale carbon dioxide. This is common in mouth breathers. The Buteyko method uses nasal breathing which results in greater levels of nitric oxide being transported into your lungs. The nasal cavities produce and contain high levels of nitric oxide which is important for proper vasodilation, nutrient and oxygen delivery.

As Patrick McKeown, author of ***'The Oxygen Advantage' and 'The Breathing Cure'*** notes, one way to learn nasal breathing is to tape over your mouth with some micropore tape. This can be done during the day or at night while you are sleeping. To avoid the tape making your skin sore, adding some coconut oil or olive oil to your lips and edges of your mouth can help. Over time, you should see your ability to breathe nasally without tape improve and your carbon dioxide tolerance should also improve. Having sufficient levels of carbon dioxide in your lungs is important because a lack of it results in blood vessel constriction and may have adverse effects on tissue oxygenation and heart function.

You can assess your current breathing volume using the Control Pause Technique.

To do this, Patrick McKeown explains that you need to first be at rest for a minimum of ten minutes. The best time to measure your breathing volume is as soon as you wake up. This is when you will get the most accurate result and you cannot influence your breathing during sleep.

To measure your Bolt Score using the Control Pause method (CP), take a small silent breath in through your nose and a small silent breath out through your nose. Pinch the top of your nose with your fingers to prevent any further air going into your lungs. Using a stopwatch, count the number of seconds until you feel the first signs of air hunger. As soon as you feel this, you have finished measuring your breathing volume. This is not a test to see how long you can hold your breath, but a test to see how long it takes before ***you feel the first signs of air hunger***. Your inhalation after the breath hold should not be any deeper than the previous normal breaths. If you need to take a sharp intake of breath then you have held your breath for too long.

The lower your breath hold period in seconds, the greater your breathing volume, and as McKeown explains, the greater your anxiety symptoms. He explains that big breathers are generally more stressed than breathers who take in the correct volume of air.

The goal is to achieve a CP of 40 seconds, consistently over a period of 6 months. If you are working on the Buteyko method correctly you should see an increase of approximately 3 to 4 seconds each week. A CP of less than 15 seconds is indicative of respiratory issues such as asthma, disordered breathing in sleep, and anxiety. For an example of how to test your Bolt score, listen to an interview with Patrick McKeown on my podcast, High Performance Health. In the episode, Patrick took me through the Control Pause method and measured my Bolt score. It indicated disordered breathing (most likely as a result of the asthma I experience) and so it has been something I have since been working on to improve.

McKeown explains that you should start to feel better each time your CP improves by 5 seconds.

Wim Hof Breathing

Iceman Wim Hof is a Danish yogi known for achieving intense feats of physical endurance in extreme conditions. In 2007 Wim Hof climbed to an altitude of 7,200 metres (23,600 ft) on Mount Everest wearing only shorts and shoes.

He uses a breathwork technique that teaches you to hold your breath for progressively longer periods of time. The technique involves thirty cycles of continuous breathwork with no pauses between each inhalation and exhalation. It is a form of rhythmic breathing and the exhalations should be relaxed - you are not supposed to be fully exhaling on each outbreath, but instead leaving some air in the lungs. After taking 30 continuous breaths in, fully exhale and hold your breath for as long as possible. Once you are no longer able to hold your breath, inhale and hold your breath for 15 to 30 seconds. You should repeat the process for 2-3 rounds. Wim Hof has a great app that you can download to take you through the process.

The benefits of the Wim Hof breathing technique include:

- an Increase in red blood cell production
- higher levels of nitric oxide production. Nitric oxide is involved in many cellular processes, including vasodilation - the widening of the blood vessels. This helps to increase the delivery of nutrients and oxygen to muscles and so can enhance exercise performance.
- the production of growth factors that lead to the development of new blood vessels.

SOMA Breath

We have talked about the benefits of meditation and breathwork throughout this chapter, but one of my favourite practices is SOMA Breath. This is a series of ancient pranayama breathing techniques combined with music, meditation and affirmations.

SOMA Breath was created by my friend and former podcast guest, Niraj Naik - 'The Renegade Pharmacist').

SOMA Breath guided meditations are an incredible way to correct your normal breathing rate so that at rest it is between 5 and 6 breaths per minute. On average people typically take between 12 and 20 breaths per minute. Slowing your breath to 5 to 6 breaths per minute can help protect against disease, enhance emotional regulation and help you to achieve more of a flow state.

The SOMA Breath technique can help to:

- improve your tolerance to carbon dioxide
- increase oxygen utilization
- enhance cardiovascular health, leading to better stamina, endurance and improved fitness
- balance your nervous system
- achieve a calmer, clearer mind
- reduce inflammation
- enhance your mind-body connection
- achieve a deep state of meditation
- improve mental and physical resilience.

The mild state of hypoxia induced is said to help to enhance memory and cognitive function. It may also stimulate stem cells to spur the repair and growth of new cells.

Niraj's music is beautiful to listen to and the SOMA Breath meditations can facilitate self-hypnosis so that you can reprogramme your mind and install new beliefs.

Rhythmic breathing (as used in the Wim Hof and SOMA Breath techniques) hyper-oxygenates the body, inhaling more oxygen and exhaling more carbon dioxide than normal. This has been shown to alter the pH of the bloodstream and create a strong electromagnetic field and current that flows through the body. It is a powerful way to raise your vibration and increase your ability to visualise the life that you want.i have found that over time, daily meditation and breathwork practice helps me to have a calmer and clearer mind, improved emotional regulation and better decision making.

Earlier you learned how your brain waves need to be at 19 cycles per second to achieve a flow state and that when you move into high beta, your thoughts become more erratic and agitated. Smooth consistent breathing leads to calmer, more coherent thoughts.

I remember one of the many clinical psychologists that I saw while being treated for depression, explaining to me that I was "not in control of my mind". Until he said this to me I hadn't really thought much about what being in control of my mind meant. ***My mind just was.*** Those sessions lead to me using cognitive behavioural therapy (CBT) practices to try and understand what my thoughts were. I learned to question thoughts and whether they were based in reality. If you're familiar with CBT you'll understand that part of the process is questioning your thoughts and whether you know them to be absolutely true. That was the beginning of my journey and understanding that I needed to master my mind if I wanted to escape the mental torment and anguish that came alongside depression.

Since then I have studied various breathwork and meditation practices in my quest to master my mind. What I have learned is that looking after your mind is no different to looking after your body. It is a daily practice. Just as you need to move your body to keep it strong, you need to exercise your brain in a way that strengthens your mind and your soul.

Whether or not you are religious, one thing seems clear - we are all on a spiritual path to enlightenment. Practices such as breathwork, meditation and gratitude give us access to higher levels of depth, clarity and flow.

Our breath and our brain waves are the entry point to our subconscious mind and all its riches. It is the place from which we can create our best version of ourselves and our ideal reality. It liberates us.

The hypoxic breathwork techniques used in SOMA and Wim Hof breathing are forms of hormesis - a low dose of stress that is applied to the body to stimulate a positive stress response. It does this by turning on your survival mode, similar to the way that saunas, cold thermogenesis and fasting do. I discuss how these practices can enhance your longevity and performance in the next chapter.

For more information on SOMA Breath and the other techniques outlined in this chapter, go to www.rethinkhealth.club.

BOX BREATHING

Box breathing is a technique commonly used by US Navy Seals to quieten the mind during periods of extreme stress. Box breathing helps to regulate the autonomic nervous system and calm you down. In box breathing you breathe in for 4 seconds, hold for 4 seconds, breathe out for 4 seconds and then exhale for 4 seconds.

I have seen improvements in both heart rate variability and sleep with clients that practice box breathing. It is a great tool for clearing your mind.

4, 7, 8 BREATHING

This involves breathing in through your nose for a count of 4, holding your breath for a count of 7 and then exhaling through your mouth more forcibly with a "whoosh" sound for the count of 8. This should be repeated a minimum of 4 times to induce a state of relaxation. This style of breathing has been shown to increase GABA (Gamma Aminobutyric Acid) - an inhibitory neurotransmitter that is essential for the proper functioning of your brain and central nervous system. It has the effect of reducing excessive brain activity and promoting a state of calm.

NADI SHODHANA: ALTERNATE NOSTRIL BREATHING

Alternate nostril breathing is a great way to restore balance and calm the mind and body. It is a useful tool to have when you are feeling agitated or frazzled. When you are trying to do too many things at once or are distracted by agitated thoughts, you are energetically, out of alignment.

Alternate nostril breathing has been shown to:

- calm our minds and lower stress
- improve our ability to focus the mind
- restore balance in the left and right hemispheres of the brain
- clear the energetic channels
- rejuvenate the nervous system
- remove toxins.

If you are feeling stressed at work, have a performance related worry about a forthcoming presentation or event or simply want to relax, alternate nostril breathing can really help to bring you back in alignment and centre your body and mind. If you are someone who finds meditation difficult with a mind that won't settle, doing some alternate nostril breathing before can help. Here's how to engage in alternate nostril breathing:

1. Sit in a comfortable position with your spine upright and your shoulders back and down.
1. With your dominant hand (right or left hand), bring your index finger and middle finger to rest between your eyebrows to use them as an anchor.
1. Close your eyes and take a deep breath in and out through your nose to prepare.
1. Close your right nostril with your right thumb. Inhale through the left nostril at a slow and steady pace.
1. Close the left nostril with your ring finger. Both nostrils should be closed. Hold your breath for a brief pause.
1. Open your right nostril and release the breath slowly through the right nostril. Pause briefly at the bottom of the exhale.
1. Inhale slowly through the right side.
1. Hold both nostrils closed briefly.
1. Open the left nostril and release the breath slowly through the left nostril. Pause briefly at the bottom
1. Repeat the cycle 5-10 times.

This breathing should be done mindfully - allowing your mind to follow the inhales and exhales.

Steps 5-9 represent one complete cycle of alternate nostril breathing. If you're moving through the sequence slowly, one cycle should take you about 30-40 seconds. Move through 5-10 cycles when you're feeling stressed, anxious, or in need of a reset.

Consistency is helpful, so try to match the length of your inhales, pauses, and exhales. For example, you can start to inhale for a count of five, hold for five, exhale for five, hold for five. You can slowly increase your count as you refine your practice.

While many of the techniques I have identified above utilise the power of the mind and the breath to mediate stress, there is a physical stressor that we are all exposed to in modern society that is invisible, but is becoming more profound. That stress is from electromagnetic field radiation ("EMF").

EMF RADIATION

Over the last 100 or so years, we have had an explosion in our use of electronic technology. The United States alone has over half a million miles of high-voltage power lines. We have tens of millions of broadcasting transmitters, hundreds of millions of screens from laptops and television screens and radiation from WiFli networks and mobile phones all around us. Humans are all electromagnetic beings and are being constantly bombarded with environmental pollution in the form of electromagnetic frequency radiation (EMF). The sensitivity of individuals to EMF varies and not all people experience symptoms as a result of it. Nonetheless, here is a list of issues that have been associated with EMF:

- headaches and vision problems
- mood disorders in the form of irritability, depression, loss in motivation and anxiety
- disturbances to sleep and fatigue
- fertility issues
- lowered physical performance.

The effects of EMF radiation can be magnified by metallic objects such as:

- those that we carry or wear - keys, jewellery, watches, mobile phones; and

- those in our offices and homes - water and gas pipes, electrical circuits

Metallic objects can act as antennae and magnify these energy waves and potentially alter the natural balance of our body's biochemical patterns.

There have been over 30,000 studies on the health effects of EMF. Children absorb twice the amount of radiation as adults (and their bone marrow absorbs up to ten times more). Children's skulls are also thinner than adults.

While going into extensive detail of EMF is beyond the scope of this book, be mindful that if you want to optimise your health and performance and limit your risk of chronic disease, you should at the very least take a few measures to limit your exposure:

- Reduce the number of EMF sources in your home and office. Keep electronics out of your bedroom and minimise the use of smart devices and appliances.
- Use wired accessories instead of bluetooth, such as wired headphones where possible.
- Keep your phone twelve inches away from your face or chest. If your phone is in your bedroom at night, either turn it off or turn it to airplane mode.
- Limit time spent on devices as much as possible.
- Use an EMF protector shield such as Defender Shield to help reduce EMF frequencies from reaching your body.
- Use dirty electricity filters in the main rooms of your home.
- Ensure that you have good mineral status. EMF increases calcium channels to open in the brain which then increases susceptibility to headaches, irritability, fatigue and insomnia. Magnesium is a natural calcium channel blocker and so optimising levels of magnesium may help to reduce damage from EMF.

- Connect to an ethernet cable as much as possible rather than using wifi.
- When not using the wireless router, unplug it or switch it off. At the very least do this at night so that you are minimising EMF while your body is resting and repairing in sleep.
- Avoid using your phone when the signal is weak as this amplifies EMF.
- Consider wearing EMF-protective clothing when flying or exposed to high amounts of EMF.

GROUNDING AND EARTHING

Grounding is a good way of releasing accumulated positive ions from your body. Grounding or earthing is the practice of exposing your body to the natural magnetic frequencies produced by the earth. To engage in grounding, all you need to do is walk barefoot or sit on the grass, sand or even the concrete outdoors. These surfaces are conductive and the earth's energy flows through them and into our bodies, exposing us to negative ions. Excess positive ions can disrupt cellular metabolism and also increase inflammation.

Another way to engage in grounding is to stand or swim in lakes, rivers or the sea.

You can also ground by wearing grounding shoes such as the brand Earth Runners, use grounding mats under your desk and/or sleep on grounding sheets or mats, using pulsed electromagnetic devices that emit the same frequency as the earth, such as Earthpulse or Flexpulse.

The Earth is full of antioxidants that help our body to achieve equilibrium at the cellular level.

LIGHT

Light has a powerful effect on human biology. In Chapter 2 (on sleep) I explained how light can disrupt your circadian rhythm and sleep, but many people are unaware of the potential for artificial light to damage your wellness.

Exposure to artificial light has been linked to numerous diseases, including:

- cataracts
- age-related macular degeneration
- breast cancer
- metabolic disorders
- cardiovascular disease
- sleep disorders.

Over recent years, LEDs (light-emitting diodes) have replaced many other forms of bulbs. Unlike incandescent and halogen lights, LED lamps are a form of digital lighting. LED lights often have a colour changing system that allow you to dim or adjust the colour of the lights. They also have a lot of flicker which can irreparably damage the photoreceptor cells in the retina and result in headaches, lack of focus, brain fog, poor eyesight and sleep disruption. Compact fluorescent lamps can cause similar issues alongside inducing oxidative stress damage that can affect the eyes and photoreceptors on the skin.

Light can also affect metabolism in a significant way. A master regulator in our cells is mTOR which facilitates protein synthesis and growth. mTOR is activated by natural light. You can see evidence of this through growth of plants in summertime, but also in tiny humans too - have you ever noticed that your kids grow more in summer!

mTOR inhibits the recycling of damaged cells and so you need darkness too for your other master regulator, AMP-activated protein kinase (AMPK) to stimulate the recycling of cellular materials.

If you are constantly exposed to light, you spend more time in mTOR activation (in growth and anabolism). In excess, this is associated with cancer and a shorter life span. This can also happen if, like many people in modern society you are constantly eating for 16 hours or more per 24 hour period. In short you need to balance mTOR activation with AMPK to optimise your health and longevity.

PHOTOBIOMODULATION

Photobiomodulation therapy is the use of non-ionizing, non-thermal light treatment. It has multiple uses and when applied in the correct dose and at the correct wavelengths can reduce pain, alleviate inflammation and stimulate tissue healing and regeneration. Depending on the type of therapy, it can use many different wavelengths of light including UV light, blue light, green light, near-, mid- and far-infrared wavelengths.

Not all light is visible to the naked eye.

THE BENEFITS OF RED LIGHT

Visible red light consists of light wavelengths in the 600-750nm. Near infra-red light ranges between 700nm and 1200nm. In the higher ranges, near-infrared light penetrates deep into the body and has been shown to stimulate mitochondrial pathways that assist with ATP production. It does this by interacting with a photoreceptor called cytochrome c oxidase. Red light also creates a temporary, low-dose metabolic stress. This type of stress is known as hormesis, which (as previously mentioned) is also a primary mechanism behind why exercise works. It essentially builds up the anti-inflammatory, anti-oxidant and cell defense systems of the cell. It also enhances the release of nitric oxide.

Numerous scientific studies have shown the benefits of red light therapy for improved recovery after exercise. Olympic athletes often use red light therapy to increase time to exhaustion. Red light therapy has been shown to stimulate stem cells, increase muscle blood flow and increase the speed of regeneration in ligaments and tendons.

Red light therapy for Anti-aging

Red light therapy is also a useful biohack for looking younger. You may have heard of red light facials which can help to regenerate the cells in your face, fade fine lines and reduce wrinkles.

Red and near infrared light are getting incredible results in the anti-aging communities and dermatologists and plastic surgeons are capitalizing on the benefits of red light for anti-aging. Red light therapy is a safe and welcome alternative to more invasive procedures such as botox injections and surgeries to rejuvenate skin. This is because red light powerfully stimulates both collagen and elastin production. It has been shown to eradicate lines and wrinkles, as well as the appearance of scars, acne, cellulite, surface varicose veins.

A review by Harvard Professor Michael Hamblin has found that red and near-infrared light therapy can:

- Lessen the signs of damage to the skin including DNA damage and damage from UV light
- Reduce wrinkles
- Enhance both collagen synthesis and collagen density. In fact, research has shown it can enhance production of collagen by 31%. This is really important as it is the loss in collagen that is in part responsible for the saggy skin that can come with aging including around the neck and jowls.

- Accelerate repair in the epithelial layer of skin and also combat other skin conditions like acne, hyperpigmentation, keloid scarring, vitiligo and psoriasis. It has been shown to speed up the healing of wounds by enhancing skin tissue repair and growth of new skin cells.

I personally use my clinical grade red and near-infrared light at home daily, to enhance my energy and improve skin and muscle health.

Red Light Therapy and Hair Growth

Red light can also be used to enhance hair growth.

Red light has proven to help both women and men with various conditions to regrow hair and even thicken the diameter of individual hair strands. It has been shown to help women with alopecia to significantly regrow and thicken hair and also to regrow hair in men with hair loss in several studies. LLet me give you a little bit of information on how hair growth works.

Essentially hair growth takes place in several phases:

- Anagen—which is the growth phase
- Catagen—which is when the hair transitions upwards towards the skin pores and
- Telogen— when the dermal papillae (area of blood supply) fully separate from the hair follicle. After around 5-6 weeks the dermal papillae moves upwards to meet the hair follicles again and the hair matrix starts forming more hair. This is when it goes back to the anagen phase.

Red and near-infrared light has been shown to help transition hair from the telogen phase back to the anagen phase and also prolong the anagen phase which is the growth phase.

It has also been shown to increase the rate of growth in the anagen phase while preventing premature catagen phases. Essentially, red light therapy helps hair stay in the growth phase, grow more, and then also re-enter the growth phase (instead of dying off). The end result is less hair loss, more hair growth and thicker fuller hair.

Research shows the benefits of red and near-infrared light therapy at different wavelengths for a range of conditions, including acne, Alzheimer's disease, arthritis, cognitive performance, depression, exercise performance, eye health, hair growth, muscle energy metabolism, pain treatment, skin rejuvenation and wound healing.[48]

There are also other benefits which have not been fully confirmed by scientific research yet, but are worth mentioning. These include increased testosterone, improved fertility, improvements in bone health, a reduction in hypertension and multiple sclerosis.

Red light therapy has been shown to have a biphasic dose, meaning that It has been clinically shown that beneficial effects are experienced from 1 minute to approximately 20 minutes. After 20 minutes, the benefits begin to decrease again like a bell curve. It is not quite understood why.

INFRARED SAUNA

Infrared sauna combines heat and light using a range of infrared therapy (depending on the sauna) and in particular, far-infrared. This is a source of radiant heat, the same type of heat that you get from the sunlight. Radiant heat directly heats objects via a process known as conversion without heating the air around the object. Far-infrared saunas heat you up from the inside as

48 https://redlightrising.co.uk/which-wavelengths-work?gclid=Cj0KCQjwirz3BRD_ARIsAImf7LMqdLFu1v_CGczPaVeXoEukAXLLc8-GyH-x6CcBmgCtZ6ojX_vg1AYaArv2EALw_wcB

well as the outside and have a more pronounced hyperthermic effect. The benefits of infrared sauna include:

- increased blood flow
- enhanced immunity
- raised white blood cell count
- improved detoxification
- better sleep
- improved hyperthermic conditioning which can help to increase muscle hypertrophy (as a result of increased net protein synthesis through the induction of heat shock proteins, increased growth hormone and improved insulin sensitivity).

Intermittent exposure to heat induces a hormetic response, which as you learned earlier provides a protective stress response. Heat exposure promotes the expression of a gene called heat shock factor 1 and subsequently heat shock proteins (HSPs) involved in stress resistance.

In flies and worms, brief exposure to heat treatment has been shown to increase their lifespan by up to 15%. Studies show that this effect is specifically mediated by HSPs[49].

Hyperthermic conditioning has also been shown to have positive effects on the brain, including:

- Increasing the storage and release of the hormone and neurotransmitter norepinephrine, which improves attention and focus.
- Increasing the hormone prolactin, which improves the speed of brain function faster by enhancing myelination and helps to repair damaged neurons.
- Raising BDNF which causes the growth of new brain cells. This improves the ability for you to retain new information.

49 https://pubmed.ncbi.nlm.nih.gov/9008657/

It may also ameliorate certain types of depression and anxiety.

- Causing an increase in dynorphin which results in increased sensitivity to the ensuing endorphins.[50]

The bottom line? The results of far-infrared saunas are so far reaching that they are definitely an important part of any plan to live younger for longer. When buying a sauna, look for a brand such as Sunlighten which have low-EMF. Saunas can also be surprisingly portable and affordable. Sunlighten supplies a good range of portable, low EMF saunas. For more information on saunas and red light therapy devices, go to www.rethinkhealth.club.

50 Source: Dr Rhonda Patrick, https://tim.blog/2014/04/10/saunas-hyperthermic-conditioning-2/#fn-11990-28

RETHINK > > >

TRADITIONAL THINKING:

- Modern life is stressful and 'being busy' is an everyday part of life.
- Stress is bad for our health.
- We need to keep pushing in order to achieve high levels of success.
- There isn't time for recovery if you want to be productive.

RETHINK:

- Not all stress is bad.
- Our perception of stress is key to how it affects us.
- Recovery cycles are key to both enhanced health & longevity and higher performance.
- Stress reduction techniques in this chapter can be used to offset the biological, environmental, mental and physical stressors that we experience in modern life.
- Some forms of stress - in the form of hormesis - can be used to:
    - enhance resilience
    - protect our health
    - become more resilient
    - become stronger in body and mind; and
    - enhance our longevity.

Chapter 6
PUTTING IT ALL TOGETHER

"Don't expect to be motivated every day to get out there and make things happen. You won't be. Don't count on motivation. Count on discipline"

Jocko Willink

If you follow the principles in this book you will be a long way towards optimizing your health and your performance and living younger for longer. You will be developing a high performance mind and body. But to really benefit you need to make health a lifestyle. As Jack Canfield says "99% is a b**th, 100-percent is a breeze".

THE POWER OF RITUALS

Rituals are fundamental to your success in health optimization and performance and longevity in business and life. If you need to think about whether or not you are going to do something you are far less likely to achieve it. If you need to think about whether or not you are going to do something you are far less likely to have locked-in consistency.

A ritual is something that is non-negotiable. You do it automatically, like brushing your teeth. Science shows that we have limited amounts of willpower and it depletes over the course of the day. We also have limited amounts of energy. Every time we have to consciously think about whether or not we are going to do something, we deplete energy.

As Jim Loehr and Tony Schwartz explain in their great book 'The Power of Full Engagement' "a ritual pulls at you...the power of rituals is that they ensure that we use as little conscious energy as possible where it is not absolutely necessary, leaving us free to strategically focus the energy available to us in creative, enriching ways."

Research shows that 95% of our behaviour is habitual. Only 5% is conscious. The more powerful we can make that unconscious and automatic behaviour, the more energy we will have to pursue our dreams and the more optimized we will become.

> One of the most powerful ways to manage your energy is to build rituals into your life that allow you to put energy-enhancing behaviors on auto-pilot. Examples of energy enhancing behaviours that improve your healthspan, your longevity and your performance that you can incorporate into your day include:

- meditation
- red light therapy
- movement - scheduled exercise and movement breaks
- fasting
- breathwork
- sleep
- reading
- journaling
- gratitude.

DAILY RITUALS

The first step is to decide which of these behaviours you are going to incorporate into your day, and when and how you will do them. You need to commit to when, where and how a behavior will happen.

For example, one of my daily practices is a 20 minute meditation every morning when I wake up.

Ritual	Meditation
When	5.30am: Straight after waking and using the bathroom
Where	In my bedroom, in front of my red light or in the sauna
How long	20 minutes
How	Vedic meditation followed by 2-3 minutes of visualisation.

I classify this as a non-negotiable. This means that I don't need to expend energy thinking about whether or not I will meditate today. I simply do it, right after waking up. It has become a ritual much like brushing my teeth.

A morning routine, a set of carefully chosen rituals that you choose to perform in the morning is one of the most powerful ways to start the day. How you start the day sets the tone for the day ahead. Many people rush out of bed, bleary-eyed after snoozing their alarms multiple times, before checking their emails or messages and beginning to respond to other people's priorities from the get-go. Your morning is a precious time and is one of the few parts of the day that you can truly control. That is why when I work with clients, we look not just at their evening routines but their morning routines.

Your morning routine should be a 'primer' for your day, priming your mind and body for a day of optimal attention, productivity, performance and success. I spent around 5 years playing around with my morning routine to find the most optimal set of rituals for me. This is what my morning routine currently looks like:

5:30am - Wake up, meditate while engaging in red light therapy/ sauna

5:55am - Hot/cold contrast shower and affirmations

6:30am - Black coffee, reading and journaling

6:45am - Fasted walk in nature with my dogs (helps with circadian alignment, fat burning and parasympathetic activity).

7.30am - Family time

8:00am - School run

8:30am - Deep work

Deep work is where I switch off my phone and emails, and work on my most important tasks of the day (my MITs). I got this idea from Leo Babauta, author of ***'Zen to Done: The Ultimate Simple Productivity System'***.

Research shows that just like our circadian rhythm we work best in cycles - 90 minute cycles to be precise. I divide my work into 90 minute blocks with a 10 minute break in between to enhance productivity. I don't work this intensively every day as I have designed my business around my children so that I can be there to watch their sports fixtures and competitions in the afternoons that they play.

NUTRITION

While I don't follow a specific dietary protocol such as the keto diet, I do keep my daytime levels of carbohydrates low. As someone who is genetically sensitive to carbohydrates I have found that eating carbohydrates during the day tends to make me feel more sluggish and experience brain fog.

The food that I eat is designed to keep my energy levels high and fuel my body to maximise my mental focus and clarity. For this reason my daily meals look something like this:

Breakfast (around 9-10am)

Breakfast is usually a higher protein breakfast such as:

- Scrambled or poached eggs with a little bit of grass fed butter and sea salt, avocado and tomatoes
- Greek style yoghurt with berries, coconut, superfood powders and some almonds
- A superfood smoothie with pea protein, wild blueberry powder, greens, fresh berries and almond butter

Alternatively I may simply fast until midday and drink an essential amino acid blend (to help maintain muscle mass and focus) or bone broth mid-morning.

Lunch (1pm)

Lunch is almost always a large salad with plenty of leafy greens, tomatoes, cucumber, broccoli, avocado, red onion, radishes and olives with a decent serving of protein such as chicken or fish. The salad is usually dressed simply in olive oil, raw apple cider vinegar and mustard.

Dinner (6.30pm)

Dinnertime is when we tend to have something more adventurous. My husband and I both love cooking and so we cook fresh food every night. Some evenings we may have something like a Thai red curry. More often than not, dinner consists of grass fed beef or lamb, free range chicken or fish with a large serving of cruciferous vegetables and a small serving of starchy carbohydrates such as coconut rice, sweet potato or new potatoes.

Eating carbohydrates at night helps me to sleep better, but I'm careful with the amount of carbohydrates I eat in the evening; just enough to help me sleep well, but not too much such that it is elevating my blood sugar. After wearing a continuous blood glucose monitor for 28 days, I found that a small serving of carbohydrates at dinner and a glass of resveratrol containing red wine (on weekends) does not particularly elevate my blood sugar.

By a small serving of carbohydrates, I mean approximately two-thirds of the size of my clenched fist. Sometimes if I've done a very heavy workout I may have a bit more than this, but generally speaking I limit my carbohydrates to that size. This amount is sufficient to satisfy me while still enabling me to stay lean and healthy and avoid the gains in visceral fat and inflammation that often occurs when blood sugar is high.

I always finish dinner at least 3 hours before going to bed (unless we are entertaining). Eating at 6.30pm gives me a guaranteed minimum overnight fasting period of 14 hours and when I skip breakfast, 16 hours.

At our family dinner we all go round the table and name one to three things that we are grateful for. We celebrate our successes of the day and talk about any difficulties or problems we have encountered.

WEEKLY RITUALS

Every Sunday I review how the previous week went, noting any difficulties I encountered and how I might improve on these. I also spend an hour or two planning my week ahead, focusing on what I want to achieve and how I will achieve it.

I spoke in more detail about the exercise that I do on a weekly basis in Chapter 3, but each week I will try and tick off the following combination of workouts:

- 3 to 5 resistance based workouts using either bodyweight or strength training
- 1-2 interval training workouts incorporating sprints, either running or on a stationary bike
- A longer endurance cardio session (around 60-90 minutes) - hiking or cycling
- A yoga session
- A foam rolling/mobility workout.

As mentioned above, I also intersperse my working day with Tabata workouts such as brief amounts of time skipping or rebounding.

I engage in red light therapy and/or sauna daily as part of my meditation practice, which gives me a healthy dose of red, far, mid and near infrared light. In addition to this, I spend as much time as I can outside, including moving my home office to the garden in warmer weather.

OTHER PRACTICES

A couple of times a year I will do an extended fasting period or detox protocol.

As regards supplementation, I cycle in and out of supplements depending on what my body needs, but there are certain staples that I always use:

- Omega-3
- B vitamins
- An antioxidant/polyphenol blend
- Magnesium
- Greens powder
- Evening primrose oil
- Vitamin D3 with K2 between October and March
- Vitamin C
- Collagen and/or bone broth
- An essential amino acid blend
- Medicinal mushrooms, such as a lion's mane or chaga
- A nootropic blend (I don't take this 7-days a week and cycle between differing varieties as otherwise due to attenuation, I find my brain quickly becomes tolerant).

FINAL NOTES

I hope that this book has convinced you of the need to take a truly holistic approach to health. The old paradigms that our health outcomes depend upon genetics, or that the way we age is linear and we have very little control over it, are not based in reality. Science demonstrates otherwise. We have the ability to signal our genes in new ways through our environment, our lifestyle, our thoughts and our behaviours.

Health optimization is a truly holistic model. It's one that requires the integration of mind, body, spirit and lifestyle. When all are aligned we feel better, show up better and can live an extraordinary life.

My own journey has shown that if you put your health on the back burner while you chase other goals, thinking that you'll come back to it later, you may face a long journey to get back on track. That is if indeed you are given the chance to do so. I feel so lucky to have been given a second chance after recovering from debilitating chronic depressive disorder and double pneumonia. I am so happy and grateful to be in a position to take care of the health of my mind, body and spirit and fulfil my mission in life to inspire others to do the same and unlock unparalleled levels of energy, vitality and performance.

What I'm inviting you to do is to make health an integral part of your lifestyle. It's the foundation of high performance - of longevity in business and in life. Many successful people including Richard Branson, Barack Obama and Ariana Huffington know better than to ignore their health. They focus on it, not because they have lots of free time to indulge, but because it makes them stronger and better at what they do.

What can initially appear to be little niggles, headaches, back pain, tiredness or gut issues are all signs from your body asking you to pay attention to it. Ignore them at your peril. While your doctor may tell you these are all merely signs of getting older or prescribe a drug to address the symptoms, it ignores the root cause. Your body will keep talking to you until you listen. Just make sure you don't leave it too late before you do.

It's not about signing up to a new workout plan or diet, an extreme fast or radical detox protocol that you do a few times a year to 'get back on track'. It's about daily practices and small incremental changes that optimise your physical and mental health and enable you to show up in the world as the very best version of you, whether that's as a leader, a creative, an athlete, a spouse, a parent or all of those and more.

I hope that this book has given you everything you need to start living your healthiest, happiest and most vibrant life. One thing I've found from working with so many individuals over the last 5 years is that you're unlikely to unlock your full potential doing this alone. To succeed, we need accountability and to push ourselves beyond where we would normally go. To assist with that, I recommend that you enlist the help of a friend or a coach who will hold you accountable and make sure you get where you want to go (or further). Whatever you do, make sure that what you've learned does not just become 'shelf help'. Take action and get started straight away. Small steps taken daily yield the biggest results.

The difference that a tiny improvement can make over time is striking. The mathematics of it shows that if you can get 1% better each day for one year, you'll end up 37 times better by the time you're done.

On the other hand if you get 1% worse each day for one year, you'll decline down almost to zero.

What starts as a small win or a minor setback grows into something much more significant. I've been down there at zero and while it's no fun, you can still get better. The body by its very nature wants to be healthy. You can become the alchemist (and not be beholden to the pharmacist) and enjoy extraordinary health.

WHAT NEXT?

After years of investment and experimentation with different biohacks and programmes, I have developed my own methodology to optimise physical, mental and spiritual health and live a vibrant life.

My team and I have done the work, we've removed the guesswork and the pain of trial and error so that you don't have to waste time and money doing so. We've uncovered the formula to fast and sustainable results - results that improve with time and grow with you.

If you would like help achieving ever greater results and become that vibrant and healthy high performer you read about in Chapter 1, head over to www.rethinkhealth.club for a free masterclass on how you can live younger, for longer.

A truly extraordinary life awaits you...

Made in the USA
Monee, IL
18 December 2021

86343919R00128